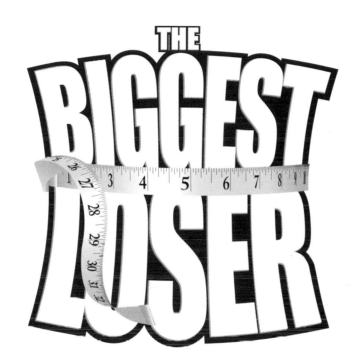

THE BIGGEST LOSER

NBC

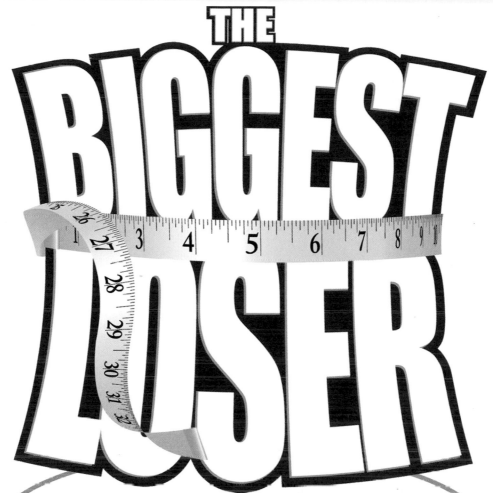

THE BIGGEST LOSER

The Weight-Loss Program to Transform Your Body, Health, and Life

—Adapted from NBC's Hit Show!

The *Biggest Loser* Experts and Cast

with Maggie Greenwood-Robinson, PhD

Foreword by Bob Harper

Printed in the United States of America
Rodale Inc. makes every effort to use acid-free ⊗, recycled paper ♻.

NBCU, Reveille, and 25/7 Productions would like to thank the many people who gave their time and energy to this project: 3Ball Productions, Stephen Andrade, Louise Braverman, Dave Broome, Brendan Carretta, Tricia Chaves, Julie Chebbi, Scot Chastain, Tami Booth Corwin, Lisa Dolin, Milissa Douponce, John Farrell, Dawn Fiore, Jodi Flicker, Kurt B. Ford, Marty Frey, John Foy, Jeff Gaspin, Linda Gilbert, Karma Goodman, Beth Goss, Marc Graboff, Erica Gruen, Cathy Gruhn, Bob Harper, Heather Halloway, Frederick Huntsberry, Allison Johnson, Helen Jorda, Allison Kaz, Loretta Kraft, Laura Kuhn, Beth Lamb, Roni Lubliner, Vince Manze, Rebecca Marks, Bob Meyer, John D. Miller, Kam Naderi, Todd Nelson, Jeanne Newman, Jennifer O'Connell, Carole Panick, Jerry Petry, LeeAnn Platner, Craig Plestis, Lisa Rafferty, Amy Rhodes, Beth Roberts, JD Roth, Troy Searer, Leslie Schneider, Ben Silverman, Ray Slay, Andrea Smith, Charles Steenveld, Lee Straus, Amy Super, Deborah Thomas, Brian Wendel, Curt Williams, Joanna Williams, Yong Yam, David Yeh, and Jeff Zucker

Product Development and Direction: Dave Broome, Cindy Chang, Mark Koops, Kim Niemi

Project Coordinators: Chad Bennett, Neysa Gordon

The recipes Spicy Breakfast Grains (page 122), Banana Fudge Smoothie (page 123), Blueberry Bran Mini Muffins (page 125), Barbecue Lentils (page 129), Icy Gazpacho (page 133), Salad Romesco (page 134), Tomato Lentil Soup (page 135), Curried Vegetable Stew (page 137), Edamame Guacamole (page 145), Creamy Hummus (page 146), Mint Tea (page 158), and Tangy Tahini Mustard Sauce (page 156) are adapted from *Stop the Clock! Cooking* by Cheryl Forberg.

Book design by Joanna Williams

Photographs by Per Bernal (photo of Bob Harper on page v, plus pages vi and 58 to 68); Mitch Mandel (pages 40, 41, 120, top left, 161, 167, 179); Kurt Wilson (pages 163, 165, 176, 180); Rodale Images (page 174); Photodisc (pages 120, bottom center and bottom right, 121, 169); Brian Hagiwara/Foodpix/Picture Arts (pages 120, top right, and 128); John E. Kelly/Foodpix/Picture Arts (page 120, bottom left); Mark Thomas/Foodpix/Picture Arts (page 146); Evan Skier/Foodpix/Picture Art (page 155); Brand X Pictures (pages 168, 173). Photos on pages 13 (after) and 108 were supplied by Lisa Andreone. All other photos by NBC Universal Photo. The illustration on page 31 is by Judy Newhouse.

Library of Congress Cataloging-in-Publication Data

Greenwood-Robinson, Maggie.
    The biggest loser : the weight loss program to transform your body, health, and life—adapted from NBC's hit show! / the Biggest Loser experts and cast, with Maggie Greenwood-Robinson ; foreword by Bob Harper.
        p.   cm.
    Includes index.
    ISBN-13 978-1-59486-384-4 paperback
    ISBN-10 1-59486-384-9 paperback
    1. Weight loss. 2. Reducing diets—Recipes. I. Biggest loser (Television network)
II. Title.
    RM222.2.G723 2005
    613.2′5—dc22
                                                  2005019943

Distributed to the book trade by Holtzbrinck Publishers

14   16   18   20   19   17   15   paperback

RODALE
LIVE YOUR WHOLE LIFE™

We inspire and enable people to improve their lives and the world around them

For more of our products visit **rodalestore.com** or call 800-848-4735

Contents

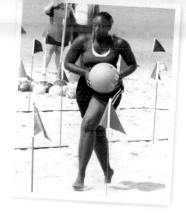

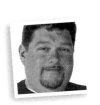
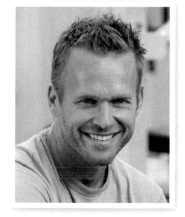
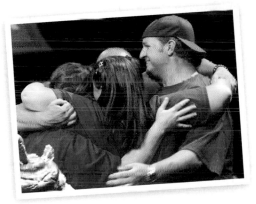
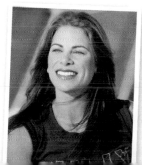

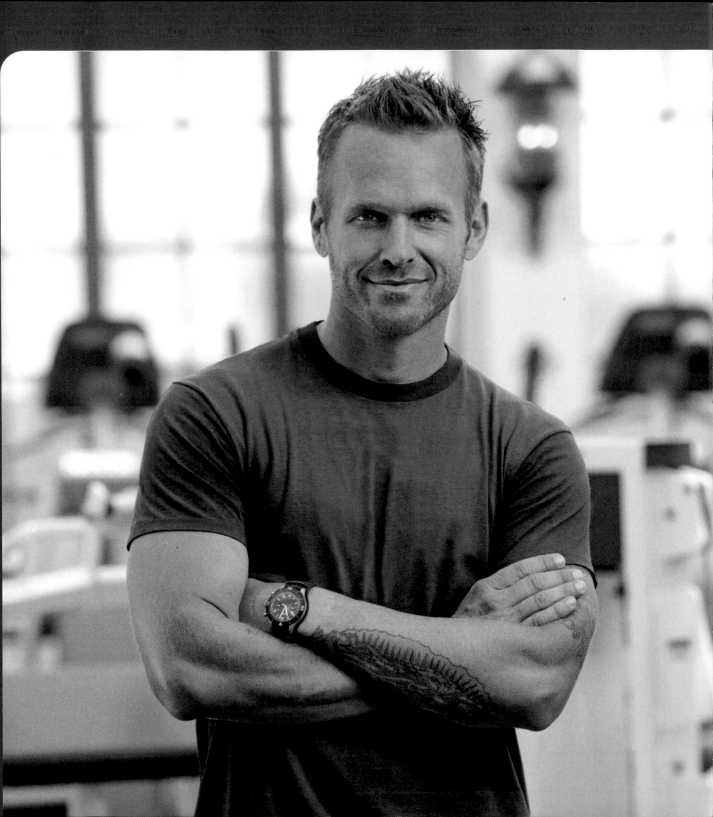

Foreword

The Biggest Loser changed my life.

When I first heard that NBC was thinking about doing a weight-loss reality show, I was naturally skeptical. I had seen all these other "makeover" shows on television that involved surgery and other extreme methods to get results, and I knew I would never morally be able to contribute my efforts to weight loss under those terms. So I went into the first meeting with my boundaries firmly in place.

Happily, I found out that *The Biggest Loser* was going to be a weight-loss show using the two best tools of all: diet and exercise. Let me tell you, my "boundary walls" came crashing down. I knew right then and there that I wanted to be one of the trainers for the show.

Then, when I first saw the contestants walking down the stairs of the ranch, my initial thought was, "Wow! I've really got my work cut out for me." I have lived in Los Angeles for more than 10 years, and I have been fortunate enough to work with some of the biggest names in this town. All of a sudden I felt like I was back to square one. What did I know? What can I teach them? Can I do this?

Well, I did—or rather they did.

If you've watched the show, you know that it involves ordinary people who need to lose a lot of weight and get control of their lives by changing their lifestyles. If you've watched the show, you know that these people lost hundreds and hundreds of pounds of weight and to this day are losing even more and keeping it off. If you've watched the show, you were naturally inspired, as I was, by seeing what these 26 people were able to do.

The book you are holding in your hands is their story—how they lost weight, how they exercised, how they changed small daily habits, and how they altered their lifestyles to become new people, inside and out. As you read their personal stories, you will be inspired by the process they lived, moved by the determination they showed, and empowered by their newfound belief in themselves. You will see yourself in these people; you will see your best friend, husband, wife, brother, sister, boyfriend, or girlfriend, and you will relate to their struggles and be inspired by their success.

This book is unlike any other "diet" book you'll ever read. Its power is that it is not a program from a diet or fitness guru; it is the collective voice of people just like you, along with me as one of their trainers, who now know from their hearts what it takes to win the weight-loss game once and for all. You'll learn their "secrets" about how to eat, how to exercise, how to stay the course, and how to be a biggest loser yourself, without resorting to crazy diets that involve suffering and sacrifice.

I'm personally thrilled to see this book in print. If the moment of truth has come for you, that you've got to take charge of your weight once and for all, you have made the best purchase of your life. Who better to guide you to a trimmer, healthier body than these 26 people, who have been so successful at what so few can seem to accomplish over the long term?

These people have shown me how important it is to stay on track. They have shown me that every single day matters. Most important, they have shown me that I have to live every day to its fullest and take everything I can out of a day because that's what they've been doing every single day.

Let me close by saying that for me this experience—working on the show and with this book—has been like no other that I've ever had. It has reignited the passion for what I do. I can't wait to get to work and share that passion. I wake up every day with a renewed purpose and a renewed focus in life. I love my job more than ever, and I owe it to my new best friends, the cast members of *The Biggest Loser*. Because of these extraordinary people, my life is forever changed. And I hope yours will be, too.

Bob Harper
Los Angeles, California

Preface

This isn't just any weight-loss book. What you're holding in your hands is a state-of-the-art, medically sound, ambitious lifestyle modification program based on the wildly successful approach we developed for *The Biggest Loser* television show. Adapted for home use, we designed this empowering, no-nonsense approach especially for those of you who are striving for a life-altering change and a dramatic weight-loss result. The kind of result that reminds your doctors, neighbors, friends, and family what lifestyle change can really accomplish. The kind of result that reverses medical problems and leaves you in need of a new wardrobe. The kind of result you wanted from other, less ambitious programs that failed to let the "new you" shine through.

When designing this dietary program, the show's weight-loss, nutrition, and fitness experts unanimously agreed that the best approach to maintaining an optimal caloric intake is to eat generous amounts of healthy low-fat protein and high-fiber vegetables and fruits. We designed this eating strategy for use in the everyday world, and while it requires discipline and some willpower, it does not require perfection, and it is by no means unrealistic. If it seems like we combined the strengths of a variety of successful eating strategies to create a novel approach, then your instincts are correct. If you are pleased with the simplicity of our formula, then we share your sentiments. Our specific dietary recommendations and formula can be found in Chapter 3.

When it comes to getting results, the principal lesson I've learned from my research and clinical experience with diets and weight loss is this: Your results depend almost entirely on how closely you follow your diet and exercise plan. If you are fully committed to following this plan to the letter, the sky is the limit. If you approach it half-heartedly and aren't willing to fight for it, your results will be modest and short-lived. Everyone who maintains a significant weight loss today does so because of their concerted daily effort and commitment to their own good health. If you're ready to lose the weight for the last time, then it's time to face the daily compromises that are weighing you down, see them for what they truly are, and decide whether they own you or you own them. If you're ready to make the permanent commitment to transforming your life, you'll find that the path we show you here is straight and true.

Everyone wants you to succeed, including your doctor. We urge you to make your doctor one of your strongest allies in this endeavor by discussing your weight-loss, dietary, and exercise goals with him or her. And my advice to doctors and other primary care providers: Never forget that the right foods and exercise are among our most powerful disease-preventing modalities. But their effectiveness, and the extent to which your patients embrace the necessary lifestyle changes, depends on your own attitude and enthusiasm when discussing these issues. When doctors and patients work closely together, the best possible results are inevitable.

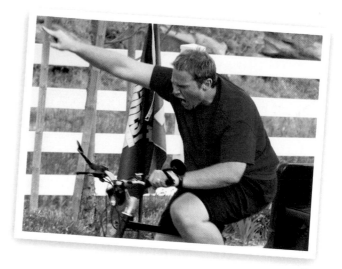

And lastly, if you ever need a reminder of the power and potency of positive lifestyle change, just view a single episode of *The Biggest Loser* TV show or read any of the inspiring personal stories within this book. Doing so is certain to spark the flame that motivated you to lose weight in the first place. I have such great respect and admiration for everybody out there who has taken the plunge and given it their all—they are role models for all of us. Talk to everyone and anyone you can find who has learned how to keep the weight off. Listen to their stories, learn from their experiences, and use this book to follow their lead. You know you'll succeed once you decide you'll never give up trying. I wish you great success and excellent health for many years to come!

Sincerely,

Michael Dansinger, MD

Michael Dansinger, MD
Weight-Loss, Nutrition, and Fitness Team, *The Biggest Loser*
Director, Tufts Popular Diet Trial
Tufts–New England Medical Center
Boston, Massachusetts

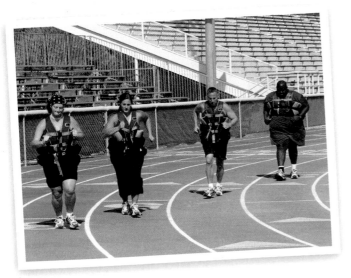

Acknowledgments

This book has been a wonderful team effort, in which I played but one part. Coaching our team was Amy Super, associate editor at Rodale, who kept the book on target, provided superb editing and suggestions, managed the project with finesse, and helped us all gel as a productive team. Chad Bennett at Reveille was our star quarterback. He was delightful to work with, a real expert at managing and facilitating what needed to get done, plus he has such a wonderful, positive attitude all the time. Mark Koops, SVP Creative Affairs of Reveille, had his heart invested in this project from the beginning, and we all felt his dedication. Cindy Chang at NBC Universal was so fast and efficient at coordinating every aspect of the project and so encouraging to all of us who were trying to meet tight deadlines. She is a real powerhouse. Thanks also go to Kim Niemi and Neysa Gordon from NBC Universal and to Dave Broome and Yong Yam from 25/7 Productions for helping every step of the way.

This project was fortunate to have on the team two extremely accomplished and credentialed experts, Dr. Michael Dansinger, MD, and Cheryl Forberg, RD, who worked with us on the nutrition and medical portions of the book and created an eating program that people everywhere can truly live with. Cheryl also kindly supplied many of the recipes for the book, which were adapted from her cookbook, *Stop the Clock! Cooking*.

Bob Harper, the celebrity trainer you see on the show, was extremely gracious with his help and time. His know-how and insight added so much substance and value to this book.

Special thanks go to Tami Booth Corwin and Erica Gruen from Rodale, who saw the potential in a book like this and made the project happen from the very start. Thanks to Joanna Williams for designing a beautiful book.

I would also like to personally thank Whitney Bell and Amber Bell, my production assistants, who helped me get my work done, and my agent Madeleine Morel for her help.

Finally, I would like to thank from my heart the cast members of seasons one and two. You are amazing and a source of personal inspiration to me. Even after 20 years of being in the fitness and writing business, I found new motivation and stronger resolve from talking to you and listening to your stories. You have given Americans everywhere hope that not only is obesity something that can be conquered, but that lives can be changed for the better in the process.

Maggie Greenwood-Robinson, PhD
Dallas, Texas

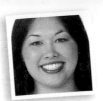
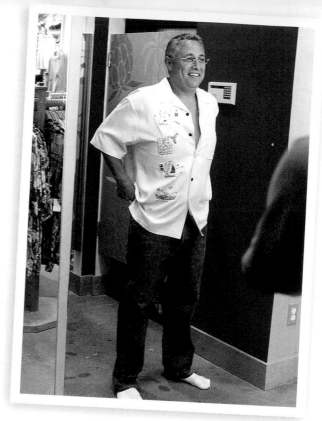
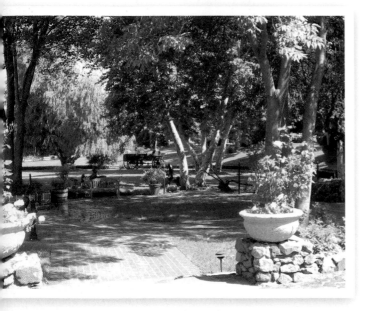
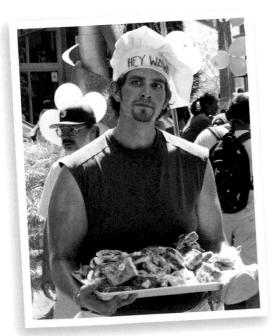

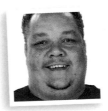
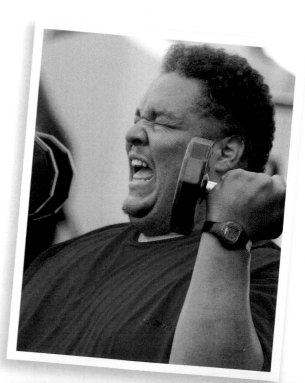

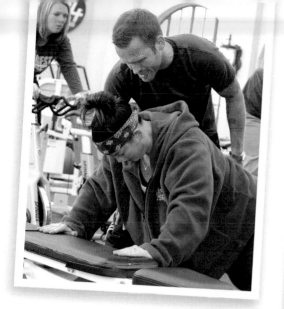
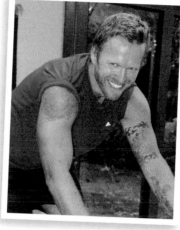
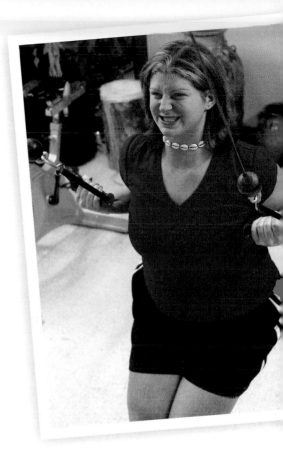
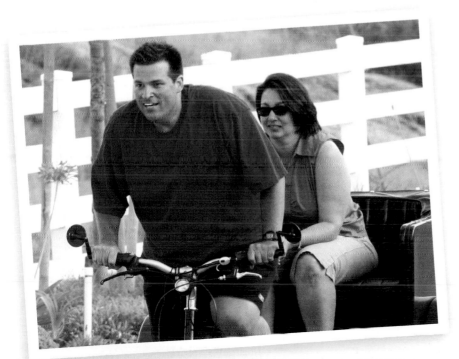
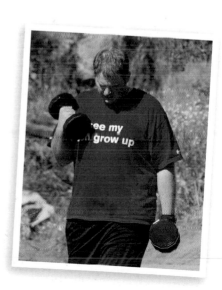

You Can Be
A BIG LOSER

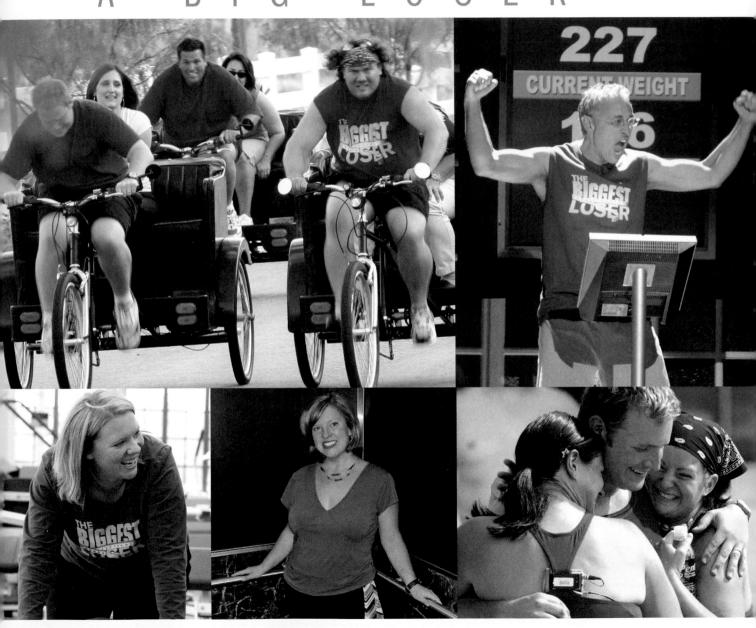

Wouldn't it be wonderful to have the body you want—slender, toned, fit, and healthy—and have it for life?

Of course it would. That's a dream shared by millions of overweight Americans, but a dream that seems elusive and impossible. Dieting works, but it doesn't usually keep weight off for good. After all, who wants to feel deprived all the time and give up enjoyable foods? Exercise isn't always fun, either; sometimes it feels like downright punishment. Sure, there's plenty of weight loss advice out there from diet gurus and so-called fitness experts. But who's right, really? And who has the solution that will work for you?

Rather than figure out the answers, try the latest diet fad, or sort out the advice from the experts, maybe the right path for you is to get down in the trenches with real people just like you who have been there, done that, and now have the bodies to prove that losing weight—and keeping it off—can become reality.

Yes, *reality.* Now you can drop those all-too-visible extra pounds by following the examples, the strategies, and the tips and tricks of real-life people who had hundreds of pounds to lose—and did it, really did it.

Who are these people who succeeded where most never do? They're the cast members of NBC's hit unscripted show, *The Biggest Loser.*

In this inspirational series, now in its second season, overweight people from all walks of life compete to lose weight through diet, exercise, and lifestyle changes. They are sequestered on a posh California ranch, where they must endure daily workout regimens, food temptations that involve overstuffed platters of high-calorie comfort foods and candy-filled dishes located at every corner—and each other.

Divided into two teams, everyone publicly weighs in on a scale at the week's end to determine which team has collectively shed the most weight. The team that loses the least weight must vote off one of its members, who is then sent packing. The dismissed cast members are charged with going back to their lives to lose more weight with the many tools and techniques they learned on the ranch. The last contestant remaining is crowned the Biggest Loser and walks away with not only a trimmer, healthier body but also prize money of $250,000.

Remember the last time you saw a friend or relative who had slimmed down so beautifully that you just had to stop and say, "What happened? How did you lose so much weight?"

Weren't you inspired by their success? And didn't you want their "secret" so you could do it, too?

The book you're holding in your hands is not the story of one successfully slender person, but of 26! These 26 people worked with the country's top fitness trainers, doctors, and nutritionists on a program that not only will slim you down, but will help you lower your cholesterol, decrease your blood pressure, strengthen your body, make you feel and look more youthful, give you more energy, and help you take control of your life. No matter how many times you've tried to lose weight in the past, no matter how many diet failures you've undergone, this book is your guide to doing it right, doing it well, and doing it permanently.

Before you get started on your new body, let's get acquainted with the people who will guide you on your journey—the 26 cast members of *The Biggest Loser.*

Season One

In season one, cast members were divided into the Red Team and the Blue Team. During production, the cast lived on a Malibu ranch stocked with food temptations—not to be cruel, but to make it more like the real world.

The Red Team

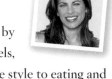

The Red Team was shepherded by celebrity fitness trainer Jillian Michaels, who brought a work-harder, lose-more style to eating and exercising.

Lisa Andreone

Overweight since childhood, Lisa was so sickly that her parents had to take out special supplemental medical insurance because of her frequent illnesses. As an adult, she considered gastric bypass surgery as a last resort but couldn't bring herself to do it, especially since she knew some people who had had the procedure but had not lost an ounce of weight. Lisa realized surgery wasn't the answer for her. Her main motivation to lose weight wasn't to be able to prance around in a thong bikini, although that was an incentive. Her motivation was fear. "I was afraid of dying of heart disease, the number-one killer of women. I didn't want to die young."

Ryan Benson

Ryan, who grew up overweight, was a closet eater. Anytime he'd be in the car by himself, he would stop at a convenience store or fast food joint and stock up on food—chili cheese dogs, hamburgers, shakes, snack pies, or doughnuts. When no one was looking, he would indulge. His wife started wondering why Ryan was gaining so much weight. After all, he didn't seem to eat that much. "I had to come clean," he said. "I actually went to therapy for a little bit, but other than that I didn't really talk about it with anyone."

Food was a negative force in his life, and he viewed exercise as a demon. By the time he was 36, Ryan had reached 330 pounds. He knew he had to change his life, or else.

Lizzeth Davalos

For Lizzeth, her turning point came after witnessing the side effects her sister endured after having gastric bypass surgery. "She started losing hair and gaining back her weight. It was bad. I didn't want to go down that path."

What needed surgery in Lizzeth's own life were her eating habits. She was a self-confessed fatty foods junkie. "I couldn't stay on healthy foods very long. After 3 days of eating healthy foods, I'd start craving pizza or other bad stuff, so I'd give in and eat it. Afterward, I'd feel so guilty. It became a vicious cycle of overeating and feeling guilty." When she reached 167 pounds on her 5 foot, 1 inch frame, her dream of looking good in a two-piece bathing suit began to evaporate.

David Fioravanti

Cheeseburgers for lunch, pizza for dinner, beer or Jack Daniels to drink, and long nights of entertaining clients helped Dave, 40, put on what felt like a ton of weight. One day he glanced in the mirror and didn't like the looks of the guy staring back.

"I was fat, and I felt like crap. I just didn't feel good about myself. I didn't want to go to the gym. I didn't even want to get dressed and go out because I didn't feel good in my clothes. I couldn't tie my shoes without losing my breath or turning purple. It was a terrible situation I had gotten myself into."

The hard-drinking, hard-partying real estate developer knew he had to make a hard change.

Matt Kamont

One of Matt's earliest childhood memories was being called "fat Matt." "I was so hurt," he recalled. "It got to the point to where I wanted to change my name. I was so sad that I told my mother, 'Please let me be named anything other than Matt. Make it Ryan, Richard, Sam—anything that doesn't rhyme with fat.'"

By high school, Matt endured more taunting and was bingeing because he felt so unpopular and unliked. "As a result, my self-esteem has never been great."

He tried several diets, but when they didn't work, he went back to his usual eating habits, gorging on comfort foods like macaroni and cheese. "When I reached 310 pounds in my mid-20s, it was the heaviest I'd ever been. I convinced myself that I'd always be heavy. I just didn't know what it was like to be thin."

Kelly Minner

More than anything, Kelly wanted to have a boyfriend, but she felt her weight was standing between her and true love. "Men judge you by your weight. If you're fat, they don't ask you out. It definitely hurts, especially if your weight is something you've struggled with all your life."

At 242 pounds, the Coopersburg, Pennsylvania, school-teacher described her dream: "To walk into a room, feel good about myself, and have men look at me and think, 'Oh my God, she's a knockout.'"

But first it would take knocking out some bad eating habits to make that dream come true.

The Blue Team

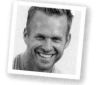

The Blue Team was led by celebrity fitness trainer Bob Harper, who focused on cast members' minds as well as their bodies, often leading his team members in meditations at the end of long hikes.

Andrea ("Drea") Baptiste

As an athlete in high school and college and a later personal trainer, Drea had to stay in top form. With her personal training profession, exercise was built into the schedule, so she stayed in shape.

But later Drea got busy with her new career as a pharmaceutical sales rep, and neither exercising nor healthy meals was a priority. She indulged in junk food and fast food and pushed exercise to the bottom of the priority list, making up every excuse in the book not to go to the gym. Before long, she was popping out of size 16 clothes. When she finally stepped on the scale, the needle stuck at 215 pounds. She knew she couldn't sit back and do nothing.

Gary Deckman

About 20 years ago, Gary, now 40, quit smoking cigarettes and gained a quick 25 pounds. Year after year, his weight crept up more and more, reaching its highest at 226 pounds. Gary was known to wolf down an entire large pizza all by himself two or three times a week and eat loads of Japanese noodles. "I basically ate anything I wanted and got no exercise."

As a result of his poor health habits, other things started creeping up on him, too: high blood pressure, high cholesterol, asthma, acid reflux disease, and bad medical reports. He had neither the energy nor the stamina to keep up with his children.

Finally, he was fed up—and scared. The family man and semiconductor salesman knew he had to lose weight, not for his looks but for his health. "When you're my age, your focus shifts from looking good in clothes to whether you want to stay alive. After all, who wants to be a good-looking heart attack victim?"

Gary knew he had to change his lifestyle. "I looked at my wife and kids and thought, 'Life is too short.'"

Dana DeSilvio

A bad relationship with a former boyfriend helped Dana pack on 20 pounds. More pounds followed—the result of poor self-esteem. "He didn't make me feel good about myself."

Finally, Dana dumped the boyfriend and got a better, more positive guy in her life, but she was left with the extra weight. Wanting to be healthy and to have kids someday helped inspire the Nashville receptionist to slim down. "I was sick of the way I looked," said Dana, 22. "I thought, 'If I don't get this under control now, then when?'"

Kelly MacFarland

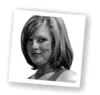

Kelly has lots of roles in life: an account manager at an insurance company by day, a stand-up comedian at night, and a food addict all the time. "My friends and I would always go out to dinner, always have drinks, and always indulge in everything."

As a child, she dreamed of being a dancer on Broadway. Those dreams were dashed as she started filling out all over and got bigger than other girls her age. "I started feeling self-conscious about my body. I would get small, then I would get big again, and then small again and big. This last time, I just got big and stayed that way."

At 223 pounds, the 31-year-old comedian had become so heavy that her stand-up act turned into a fat joke. Yet all of that weight on her 5-foot frame was no laughing matter.

Aaron Semmel

Like most fat people, Aaron knew how to lose weight. After all, he had lost the same 100 pounds over and over again by dieting and exercising. At one point, he was in such great shape that he competed in triathlons. In 2000, the skinny Los Angeles writer took some time off to travel for a year. When he returned home, so did the weight. "Starting in 2001, I gained about 20 pounds a year," he recalled. From the looks of him, Aaron had plenty of food and enjoyed it all. His weight snuck up to 261 pounds, and except for the time in high school when he weighed 300 pounds, he was in the worst shape of his adult life. Aaron wanted to run and do triathlons again, but how?

Maurice ("Mo") Walker

Raised on dishes like Southern fried chicken made by his beloved mother, Mo eventually ate his way up to 436 pounds. The Nashville-based accountant felt that his size made him unattractive to women and unattractive to employers. "Being so heavy has stopped me from getting job promotions," he said. "A lot of supervisors and managers think that because you're overweight, you're lazy and you won't work hard. It's a stereotype that won't go away."

But Mo's greatest fear wasn't losing a lady or a job promotion; it was losing his life. "My father was overweight, and he died of a stroke when I was 18. I knew I had to do something, and now was the time."

One day, Mo was standing in line at McDonald's when his cell phone rang. It was a producer telling him that he had been selected to appear on *The Biggest Loser*. He knew it was the chance of a lifetime.

Season Two

In season two, the battle of the bulge changed to become the battle of the sexes. The cast members were divided into two seven-member teams with Jillian training the men and Bob training the women. You might think such a division gives the men an unfair edge; men tend to lose weight faster than women do because most male bodies have more lean muscle mass, the driving force for metabolism. The show, however, leveled the playing field. The contestants' percentages, rather than pounds, were compared. Here's how it worked: Let's say the men's team starts at 2,000 pounds collectively, and the women's team starts at 1,500 pounds. For the men to lose 10 percent of their body weight, they'd have to lose 200 pounds. For the women to lose the same 10 percent, they'd have to lose only 150 pounds.

These cast members lived on a sprawling Simi Valley ranch, well stocked with tempting taste treats in every room.

The Red Team

In season two, Jillian applied her hard-work approach to this group of seven men.

Nick Gaza

As a stand-up comedian, Nick is a very funny guy. Unfortunately, he doesn't have much fun. Why? "Because I'm fat. There are just certain things you can't do. You can't go horseback riding. You can't go on certain rides. You can't dance as much as you want to dance."

Being a comic is only one of his talents. Nick, who began the show weighing 346 pounds, is trained as a chef and did a lot of the cooking for his team. He'd make a low-fat jam-balaya that was only 382 calories a bowl. Some of his teammates almost cheated by going back for seconds.

It's that kind of healthy cooking that will help Nick realize his ultimate goal: sticking around for another 20 to 30 years and filling them with fun.

He's on his way already. "The washcloth is reaching places it never did before."

Ruben Hernandez

The night before *The Biggest Loser* officially begins, the cast members are treated to a "last supper" of their favorite foods. Ruben Hernandez, weighing 278 pounds, dug in with both hands, literally. "By the time I was done, I felt like a disgusting pig. That feeding frenzy was exactly what I was trying to get away from," he said. "I don't want to be able to go and eat anything I want whenever I want to. This stops and it stops today."

Motivating Ruben is his old military uniform, placed strategically in his "goal closet," a display case in the contestants' workout room. "The last time I weighed what I want to weigh was when I was in the military as a paratrooper 20 years ago. Seeing that uniform really inspired me to think, 'Wow, maybe I can get back to where I was.'"

The real reason Ruben is at the ranch is because he's pushing 40, and he feels the effects of his unhealthy, inactive lifestyle. "My body can't do everything that it once did, and I don't have the energy that I once did," said Ruben, who was recently diagnosed as borderline obese.

He thinks about wanting to get married someday and raising children. He wants to be able to play full-court basketball again. He wants to wear the clothes that he used to wear but are now in his closet, gathering dust. He wants to inspire his own family to live more healthfully.

"I want to be able to do everything I want to do in life."

Matt Hoover

Being a wrestler in college burned off all the junk food and beer Matt put away on the weekends. Things got worse, though, after his athletic career was over, and Matt decided to take time off from athletics. Back surgery supplied a handy excuse to stop working out altogether. His active lifestyle became a thing of the past, and his drinking habits got out of control. He never adjusted his eating and drinking to make up for his couch-potato lifestyle, and pounds started piling on, all the way up to 340 pounds.

The 29-year-old retaining-wall salesperson from Iowa knew that his weight was affecting every area of his life. His first marriage—ironically to a fitness trainer—crumbled because he preferred the couch to the gym. His business suffered, too. "I'd go to meet with architects, engineers, or even contractors who are active and fit, and they'd see me walk in with my gut hanging over my pants. I didn't feel right; I didn't feel good about myself. When I looked and felt so bad, how could I expect others to take what I said seriously?"

Then one day, Matt happened to be watching *The Biggest Loser,* lying on the couch, with beer and chips in hand. He felt tired of lying around and knew deep down that he had the ability to change whenever he wanted to. There was an open casting call for season two in his area, and Matt answered the call.

Jeff Levine

As a family practice physician and associate professor directing women's health programs at Robert Woods Johnson Medical School, Jeff, 43, had put together a good life for himself, his wife, and his four daughters. There was only one problem, one very big problem: Food had become a drug for Jeff. It helped him stay awake. It helped him calm down. It helped him reduce stress. He had literally become addicted to food. That addiction caused his weight to climb to 400 pounds.

Eventually, it caught up with him.

"I started having a lot of physical problems. I'd get blood clots in my legs when I'd fly. I found myself falling asleep in the middle of meetings. I would joke and say I was just having 'selective narcolepsy,' that I was just bored. One time I fell asleep while talking to a patient, which was extremely embarrassing."

The health problems escalated. Jeff began to suffer very painful, obesity-related arthritis in his ankle. His blood pressure soared to dangerous levels: 160 over 90, most of the time. His blood sugars were too high, and his insulin levels were double the norm. His personal physician wanted to put him on diabetic medication.

To make matters worse, Jeff learned he had sleep apnea, a temporary suspension of breathing that occurs repeatedly during sleep and is associated with being obese. He began wearing a special face mask at night that gently pushed compressed air through his nose to keep the airway open.

These problems intruded on his quality of life. "I could no longer play basketball. I couldn't carry my kids up the stairs. When they wanted me to play soccer with them, I could play only goalie, but barely. My deteriorating health began to affect my intimacy with my wife. While you're wearing a sleep apnea mask and sound like Darth Vader, it's hard for someone to want to cuddle with you."

Jeff pictured his wife a widow—and that's when he vowed to get healthy.

Pete Thomas

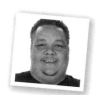

For Pete, first came love, then came marriage . . . then came 70 extra pounds, 7 years after tying the knot. Putting on weight after marriage is common for both men and women, and Pete is living proof. "Since I've been married, I've gained about 10 pounds a year. I used to play basketball recreationally, about four or five times a week. My wife asked me to cut down on my basketball and spend more time on our relationship. I cut basketball out completely and became a couch potato. I've struggled with my weight ever since."

With the middle-age milestone of age 40 looming, the 37-year-old real estate investor and mortgage broker says he wants "weight loss as a problem out of his life." He believes, "Now is the time to take care of it."

Seth Word

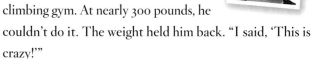

To celebrate a recent wedding anniversary, Seth and his wife went to a rock climbing gym. At nearly 300 pounds, he couldn't do it. The weight held him back. "I said, 'This is crazy!'"

Trading in his eat-on-the-run habits for regular, healthy meals hasn't been easy for this Sacramento, California, salesman, who admittedly eats to ease the stress of his 12- to 13-hour-a-day job. But he's determined. "I had to do something about my weight. I couldn't keep doing this to myself."

Seth knows losing weight will help him with his family life. "Because I work long hours, I get home, and I don't feel like doing anything. It will be different after I lose this weight. We're going to go hiking and do lots of different things in order for us to stay active and to get us away from the boob tube."

Mark Yesitis

Wake-up calls are no stranger to this 358-pound police officer from Campbell, California. Two years ago, he was diagnosed with testicular cancer and underwent radiation and surgery to remove one of his testicles. "You can just call me 'Lefty,'" he jokes.

"Until that point, I had the I'm-young-and-invincible attitude," said Mark, who has since been cured.

As the 36-year-old eyes the $250,000 prize money to be awarded to season two's Biggest Loser, he stays focused on his true goal: losing weight and getting healthier. "If you don't have your health, the money doesn't do any good."

"I beat cancer; now I'm going to beat my weight."

The Blue Team

In season two, Bob's approach catered to these seven women's minds and bodies.

Ryan Kelly

After two heartbreaking miscarriages, Ryan buried her pain in food. She began to use food as a coping mechanism. More heartbreak followed: Ryan was told she could not have children. Her weight spiraled up and up after that. Using food to get through stress became a habitual pattern that she could not break out of.

Ryan and her husband decided to adopt a little girl from Guatemala. Then to their surprise, Ryan got pregnant and was able to carry the baby full term. She was extremely happy, but she did not know how to stop bingeing when she was emotional.

Ryan tried everything to lose weight, but everything brought her back to the same point of failure. She decided that maybe, just maybe, if she had a camera in her face, she could lose weight. Ryan wrote a song to audition for *The Biggest Loser* and got on the show.

She weighed in at 225 pounds, determined to regain not only her figure but also her old confident, vivacious self.

Jen Kersey

Growing up as an overweight child was always a struggle for Jen. All of her friends were thin. Being half Asian and half white made it even harder. "In the Asian community, even if you wear a size zero, you can still be considered fat," the 24-year-old medical student explained. "I never felt like I belonged because I was always the biggest, at 5 foot 8 inches and wearing size 16s or 20s. I was teased, so I turned to food and to my studies to relieve the emotional pain."

Jen continued to gain weight during college and after she had her two children, eventually hitting 267 pounds in 2005. Now she's studying to be a physician of osteopathy, a branch of medicine that emphasizes prevention. "I know that one day I will have to tell patients to lose weight, change their eating habits, and exercise. I don't want to be a hypocrite. In order to change the lives of others, I have to change my life first."

Suzanne Mendonca

Once she started gaining weight in her teenage years, it seemed like Suzanne couldn't stop eating and putting on pounds. Many times, she'd consume 5,000 calories a day, and so the pounds piled on, even though she had always been active. "I can eat so much that it's disgusting," she said. Eventually, she ate her way up to 230 pounds.

As a 30-year-old New York City cop, Suzanne has a recurring nightmare: trying to rescue someone screaming for help, while climbing 10 flights of stairs because the elevators don't work and not being able to make it to the top.

Her weight problem has not only affected her ability to perform her job but also has jeopardized every aspect of her life. "My cholesterol reading is abnormal, my skin looks terrible, and I don't want to go out to any social occasions anymore."

One social occasion is looming: her wedding. Suzanne wants to be 100 pounds lighter before she walks down the aisle.

Shannon Mullen

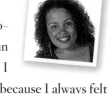

Though heavy most of her life, the 30-year-old Revere, Massachusetts, woman said, "I knew I was overweight, but I didn't think being heavy held me back because I always felt good about myself." Then she looked at her precious young daughter and did some serious thinking.

"My daughter is at the age when I started putting on all my weight," explained Shannon, who started *The Biggest Loser* weighing 257 pounds. "It's so important for me to be a role model. I've been a single mom for practically her whole life. I do everything for her. The one area I feel I'm lacking is teaching her how to eat healthy because I don't do it myself. It's hard to teach your child to do something when you don't do it well and don't have it under control."

Shannon knows that both she and her daughter will be the biggest losers in the end.

Kathryn Murphy

Growing up, Kathryn was loved with food. "In our family, food was very much connected to approval, comfort, happiness, and reward," she recalled. She was a chubby kid, and although she thinned out in high school, her weight would eventually balloon to 217 pounds.

In battling her weight over the years, the 28-year-old family law attorney from Bloomington, Minnesota, would practically starve herself, living on caffeine and cigarettes and not getting any exercise. When she felt depressed or stressed out, she'd binge in the middle of the night. "It all just added up to a huge weight gain."

A self-proclaimed overachiever, Kathryn says she usually gets results fast when she puts her mind to something. Right now, her mind is focused on getting to her goal weight of 170 pounds.

Andrea Overstreet

It was only after she gave birth to her second child that Andrea's weight problem got dangerously worse. She gained 100 pounds as a result of that pregnancy and hasn't been able to lose it since. Her weight settled at 220 pounds, and at times, she felt down on herself. Andrea, a hairdresser, believes that her clients secretly wonder how she could sell beauty without looking beautiful herself. "I know that I have a pretty face, but it is the body that needs a little work."

Andrea's other motivation to lose weight is her family. "I just want to be the best mom that I can be to my kids and help our family be more active. After I get in better shape, my husband and I will have a better sex life, too—not that it can get any better!"

Suzy Preston

Suzy spent her high school and young adult years tipping the scales at around 250 pounds. As a hairdresser, she cared more about making other people look beautiful than she did herself, even though she had a pretty face. Suzy battled her weight with diet after diet, but all she ended up with were more pounds. Then one day, she did some soul-searching about her future: "I didn't want to be single all my life. Who would want to marry a chubby girl?" That's when it hit her that eating right and being healthy had to be a way of life. She decided to put herself first and get rid of the weight that was detracting from her own good looks.

• • •

If you can relate to these stories—and you know you can—then you are about to discover how to lose every single pound of excess weight. On each page of this book, you'll go behind the scenes of *The Biggest Loser* to learn how each cast member finally got his or her weight under control.

There's really no one secret, but rather lots of secrets and strategies that, taken together, will help you get your weight under control. What you'll learn from the Biggest Losers is that losing weight and keeping it off requires a holistic approach: good nutrition, workouts that are fun, allowances for your favorite foods, and techniques to move yourself toward lifelong change.

Use this book to follow the eating plans used by the cast members, the workouts that melted off their fat, and the motivational strategies they used to stay the course. This is a book you'll want to keep by your bedside, in your kitchen, or at work—wherever and whenever you need a hefty dose of inspirational advice from people who know what it takes to be the Biggest Losers.

Now you can follow in their footsteps. Destination: a thinner, younger, and healthier you.

The journey begins on the next page!

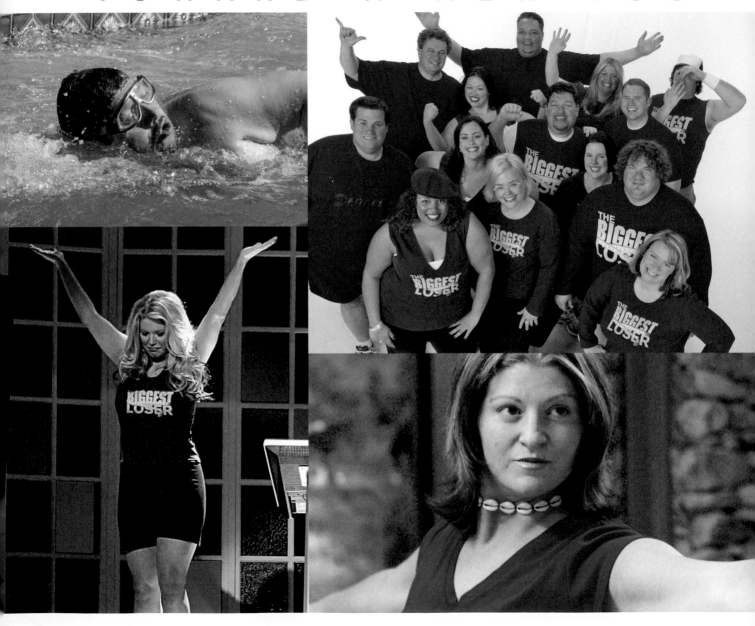

2 Getting Started
TOWARD A NEW YOU

Each cast member on *The Biggest Loser* has a different reason for losing weight—some do it for health, others for appearance, still others for psychological reasons—but all of those reasons are deeply personal.

What about you? Why do you want to lose weight?

Thinking about why you want to lose weight helps get you in the right mind-set for success. If the desire to "look better," for example, provides a strong enough motivation to shed pounds, so be it. If it's not important to you to have a beach-ready body, however, there are many other motivators that may help you stay on your weight-loss program. Let's take a look.

To Be Healthier

I didn't want to die young.
—Lisa Andreone

Like so many of the cast members, Kelly MacFarland got a blaring wake-up call: "Right before the audition for the show, I had a doctor tell me that I was not going to make it past 40 if I kept doing what I was doing and gaining weight. I'm 32; I wanted to see my 40s and beyond!"

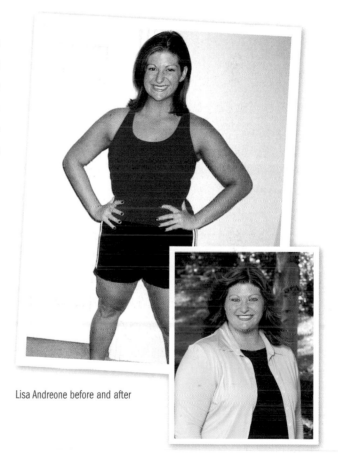

Lisa Andreone before and after

Dr. Jeff Levine had several wake-up calls. One rang out when several of his physicians insisted that he have gastric bypass surgery. He wasn't so sure.

"About a dozen of my patients have undergone successful gastric bypass surgery. The difference, though, between them and me was that they all had suffered lifelong problems with their weight. I had not. I've been overweight for about 14 years, and 10 of those years I've been obese. I didn't have a lifelong struggle with weight. I could still remember what it was like to be thin. I knew I hadn't really made a wholehearted effort to lose weight. Gastric bypass is a last resort, when you've exhausted all your options. I knew I had not exhausted all mine. That's when I knew I had to do something to save my life."

Many people want to be healthy more than they want to be skinny. One of the most important reasons to lose weight and maintain that weight loss has to do with your health. Excess weight is associated with many health problems, some of them life-threatening.

Heart disease. Heart disease is the leading cause of death in both men and women in the United States. Being overweight can have as much of an impact on your heart's health as smoking and high cholesterol, according to medical studies. It increases the risk of high blood pressure, which is associated with a risk of strokes, and promotes abnormal levels of blood cholesterol. If you sport a spare tire or a beer belly, do what you can to get rid of it: Abdominal weight is linked to an increased risk of heart disease.

Type 2 diabetes. According to the American Diabetes Association, you're at risk of developing this blood sugar metabolism disorder if you are overweight, have a sedentary lifestyle, and are over the age of 45. Uncontrolled, type 2 diabetes leads to serious medical problems, such as heart disease, kidney disease, and blindness.

Cancer. Several years ago, an important large-scale study on the relationship between cancer and obesity was conducted by the American Cancer Society. It involved 750,000 Americans from 26 states and analyzed information on the participants' body weights, smoking habits, and cancer deaths over a 13-year period, from 1959 to 1972. After adjusting for the effects of age and cigarette smoking, the study found that people whose body weight was 40 percent higher than average had an overall increased risk of cancer death—a 33 percent increase in men and a 55 percent increase in women. Overweight men had higher rates of colorectal and prostate cancers, and overweight women had higher rates of cancers of the gallbladder, breast, cervix, endometrium, uterus, and ovaries.

Osteoarthritis. This condition involves a wearing away of the tissue that protects your joints and can be both painful and debilitating. According to the Arthritis Foundation, being overweight contributes to and aggravates osteoarthritis.

Sleep apnea. With this sleep disorder, the upper respiratory airways collapse, resulting in people snoring loudly, waking up suddenly, and then returning to sleep. It causes poor sleep and severe daytime fatigue. Many overweight people are plagued with this medical condition, including Jeff Levine, and many others have borderline sleep apnea. One is Pete Thomas.

If you are overweight, losing even a little weight can help you be healthier. Medical experts generally agree that losing just 5 to 10 percent of your body weight reduces your risk of serious diseases.

To Improve Your Physical Appearance

I want to look at myself in the mirror and like what I see.

—Dave Fioravanti

Every year, millions of us embark on diets to improve our appearance. This was true for Suzanne Mendonca, who overheard people remark that she would be so much better looking if she would lose weight. "People in this world don't consider you attractive unless you have the body and the face to match," she said. It was also true of Matt Hoover, who wanted to lose weight to create a better impression on his business clients.

Generally, losing weight does make you feel more satisfied with your physical appearance. Even so, trainer Bob Harper cautioned: "The main thing is to make peace with your body now, before you try to change it. Accept where you are at the moment. Okay, you're overweight. But how great that you've decided to do something about it!"

Even if you're overweight now, you can make yourself more attractive by wearing different clothes, using makeup, having a makeover, or changing your hairstyle. The point is

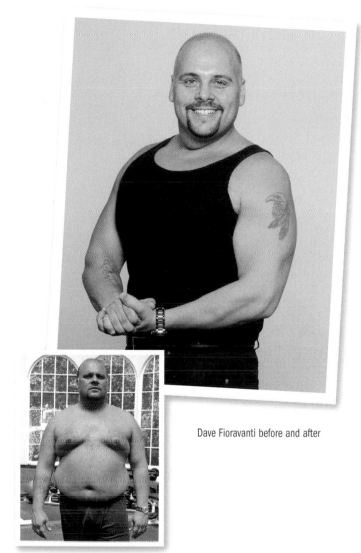

Dave Fioravanti before and after

to start feeling attractive *now* and not to make attractiveness contingent upon having a slimmer body at some point in the future.

To Look Great in Clothes

I want to fit into a two-piece bathing suit.
—Drea Baptiste

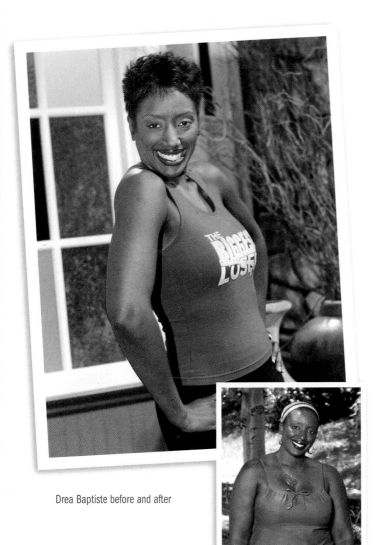

Drea Baptiste before and after

So many of the cast members expressed a desire to dress and look sexy, to shop in a greater variety of stores, and to wear cool and fashionable clothes. "When I realized that I'm not going to be able to dress the way I want because I'm too big and nothing fits me, I asked myself, 'Why should I settle for being big when I could look so much better?'" said Shannon Mullen. "At my favorite store, the largest size they carry is a 10. I'm almost double that—size 18."

Prior to coming to the ranch, Shannon bought a size 10 skirt and a medium-size top from that store. They're hanging in her goal closet, positioned strategically in front of a treadmill as a motivator. "I know that before I leave this house, I'll be able to put that outfit on," she said confidently.

The idea of wearing a two-piece bathing suit, a designer sports jacket, a sexy negligee, or a wedding dress, or just fitting into a smaller size or more fashionable clothes has a way of resuscitating the desire to lose weight. One of Suzanne Mendonca's biggest incentives for weight loss came when she got engaged and would eventually have to shop for a wedding dress. "When my fiancé and I postponed setting a date, it gave me ample time to get serious and lose weight," she explained.

When you lose weight, you expand the types and styles of clothing you can buy, as well as the number of stores at which you can buy clothes. But here's something to consider: Don't wait until you reach your goal weight to buy new clothes. Buy them over the course of losing weight. This is good for your morale and motivation and will invite compliments from other people.

To Be Fitter

I want to swim and do triathlons.
— *Aaron Semmel*

Gary Deckman, Aaron Semmel, Jeff Levine, and Mo Walker all have one thing in common, besides the need to manage their weight: They're determined never to return to the world of the unfit.

Formerly a nonexerciser, Gary now runs every day and can finally play volleyball with his kids. He also feels up to taking surfing lessons with his kids and ready to try to beat his wife at tennis. Aaron has revived his role as a triathlete. Jeff can keep up with his four active daughters. Mo can now run laps with the kids he coaches in Little League football, whereas before he could only watch from the sidelines. "Sometimes you've got to have hit bottom, like realizing you can't play tag with your kids without getting out of breath," said trainer Jillian Michaels, "before you decide to improve your level of fitness."

Among their reasons to lose weight, these cast members had a desire to become more fit. For Gary, Jeff, and Mo, this desire stemmed from wanting to do everyday activities without feeling physically taxed; for Aaron, it was a desire to take up a sport again.

Getting fit has huge payoffs and should be part of a permanent lifestyle change. Becoming fitter makes you feel athletic, helps your body burn fat and build body-shaping muscle, and improves your self-confidence and self-esteem. If you're like Gary used to be—nonactive—you need to figure out what will motivate you to get moving. If you like

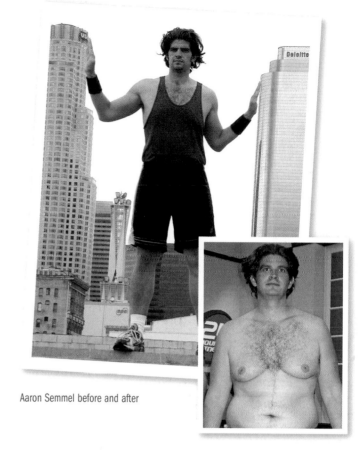

Aaron Semmel before and after

the outdoors, for example, try hiking or walking in a pleasant surrounding such as the beach, a park, or a historic neighborhood. If you're competitive like Aaron, take up a sport such as tennis, racquetball, or running.

Whatever you choose, start small—and don't think you have to devote huge chunks of time to your effort at first. "Thinking that you can't get in shape because you don't have 2 hours a day to exercise is just another excuse for doing nothing," Bob insisted. "Start small because small can only get bigger. Starting big means burning out, blowing out, getting injured—another reason you might quit altogether."

To Be Normal, without Life Revolving around Food

In my comedy act, I still talk about being obsessed with food, because I am. But I also talk about how I'm not really interested in being a size 6. I'm more interested in being strong, being able to run, and being able to squat thrust an ottoman into my car myself.

—*Kelly MacFarland*

Cast members Ryan Kelly, Kelly MacFarland, and Jeff Levine admitted to once being "addicts." Their drug of choice wasn't nicotine or cocaine; it was food. They could get strung out on food, using it to medicate themselves against stress and emotions.

To regain a sense of normalcy in her life, Ryan forced herself to get out of the house more often, away from food, and to substitute healthy activities such as exercising when she felt the urge to overeat in response to stress.

Kelly MacFarland doesn't beat herself up anymore if she goes out for drinks and dinner with her friends and overindulges; she gets up the next morning, knowing that it's a new day and a renewed chance to be active and healthy. Her advice? "Find some balance on a daily basis, so when you do have those indulgences, it's not a big deal, and you can work through them. You always have the gym and your sneakers, so if you feel like you've blown it, then you just have to work it off, and there is no guilt."

When Jeff Levine was taken out of an environment that

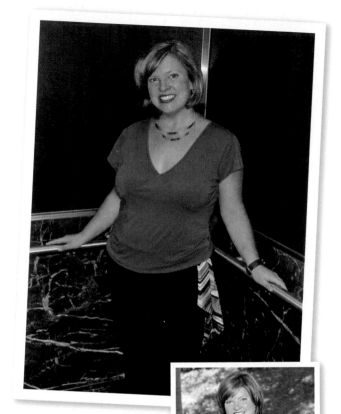

Kelly McFarland before and after

led to his food addiction and transplanted on the Simi Valley ranch, he learned one very important lesson: You can break the habits of a lifetime by changing your environment (out with the junk food, in with the health food). Make sure your kitchen and workplace are stocked with healthy choices like fruits, vegetables, lean proteins, whole grains, and low-fat dairy products. Without nutritious food on hand, you're too likely to give in to temptation or head for the nearest fast food joint or pizza parlor.

Bob Harper elaborated on this issue of living normally with food. "My clients, particularly those who have to lose a lot of weight, are often very angst-ridden when they start. They say, 'You're going to take away the food I love! You're going to make me do things I don't want to do, which is why nothing has ever worked for me!' I try to get them to relax. This isn't about beating yourself down but lifting yourself up. It involves realizing why your eating has gotten out of control and starting to think about food differently. I teach them how to work their favorite foods into their plans so they don't ever feel deprived."

As for eating in response to stress, Bob offered the following advice: "When you find yourself thinking, 'I'm going to get an ice cream cone because I've had such a bad day'—just stop. Take a moment and ask yourself, 'Am I really hungry? Do I really want this? Why do I want it?' The pause gets you thinking instead of simply acting on impulse."

Jillian added that if what you're feeling is something other than hunger, substitute a nonfood treat. "Instead of eating the ice cream, reward yourself with a manicure, massage, or bubble bath. Do something positive, healthy—something that makes you feel beautiful and is incompatible with bingeing or overeating."

To Have Better Relationships

I'd like to go to a bar and approach a guy for the first time in my life.
—Kelly Minner

Losing weight is an important thing you can do for yourself, and it does have the benefit of improving interpersonal relationships, particularly with those of the opposite sex.

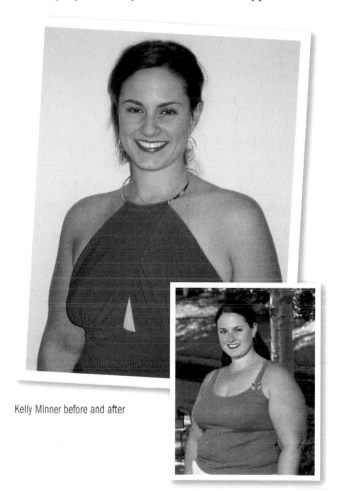

Kelly Minner before and after

Being thinner and healthier restores your sense of self-worth, a feeling often lost to being overweight, and can rebuild your capacity to feel attractive and lovable.

Mo Walker, Kelly MacFarland, Kelly Minner, and Nick Gaza each wanted to attract a mate someday but felt like their weight made them less than desirable, and oftentimes socially inactive. Married guys like Gary Deckman, Jeff Levine, and Pete Thomas all agreed that being in top form improves their intimacy with their wives.

Like buying new clothes, becoming socially more active or improving intimacy with your spouse should not be delayed until your goal weight is reached. Work on these things now.

To Gain More Self-Respect and Self-Confidence

Losing weight would help me walk around with more confidence.

— *Matt Kamont*

As the unwanted weight comes off, self-confidence builds. When you look good, you feel good, inside and out. Andrea Overstreet, for example, was teased by her brothers as a kid, and it damaged her self-confidence. Today though, she credits losing weight with boosting her self-confidence. "It has made me a stronger person. I know that I can do anything if I set my mind to it," she said.

Matt Kamont, who endured his share of teasing as a child, offered these words of encouragement if you feel de-moralized by your weight. "Just because you're overweight doesn't mean you're a 'fat-ass' or 'ugly.' It does not mean that you're worthless. You're a beautiful person who can turn your life around. Trust me, if I can do it, anybody can do it."

Kathryn Murphy had a real breakthrough in confidence building, thanks to her increased activity levels while at the ranch. "I used to feel so self-conscious about my body that I didn't want to go to the gym. I felt I was constantly being

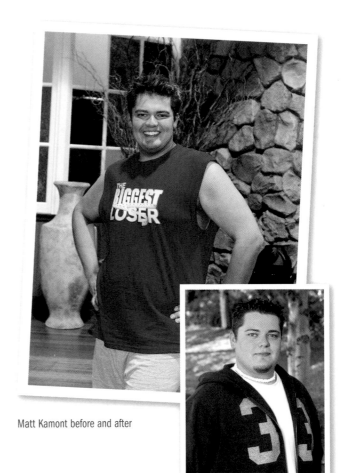

Matt Kamont before and after

judged, that I didn't belong there. Once I discovered what my body was capable of doing, I abandoned those feelings. Exercising increased my confidence."

Matt Kamont offered some additional, much-needed perspective if you're feeling low on confidence because of your weight. "About 65 percent of all Americans are fat, so the probability is that all those people who once called me 'fat' are probably fat right now, too. It's ironic, and funny, if you think about it."

There are many avenues you can take to build your self-confidence; losing weight is just one of them, but it is one that can have important benefits to you personally.

Get Organized

Before you actually begin the Biggest Loser plan, it's a good idea to get your house in order. This means organizing yourself for success so that the road to permanent slenderness and better health will be a little smoother. You know how important organization is if you've ever had to start a household project. Just think what it would be like if your tools were scattered all over your house. You'd have a pretty chaotic time trying to complete the project if you had to run from the tool shed to the garage to the backyard every time you needed a tool. To be efficient, you need to gather your tools and have them within easy reach. The same is true when you embark on something as important as losing weight. You need to get organized, with all your tools right where you need them. That said, here are the tools you need to get started.

Calorie-Counting Guide

You'll need a guide to help you keep track of the calories you're eating each day. Calorie counts of common foods are available for free on the Web. One particularly good database is the U.S. Department of Agriculture's online nutrient database at www.nal.usda.gov/fnic/foodcomp/search/.

There are also dozens of books on the market that supply the same information. Look for one that is reasonably comprehensive. The data should be arranged so that it is easy to find the foods you're looking for. In other words, the book should be "user-friendly."

You won't have to use this forever, though, because in a few weeks, you'll be able to gauge the number of calories in the foods and portions you typically eat.

Food Scale and Measuring Cups and Spoons

To help you manage your portions, these tools are a must for measuring out the exact quantities of all the food you eat. After a while, you'll know what a cup of rice or 4 ounces of meat looks like and you can stop measuring.

Food Journal

People who keep food journals tend to be more successful at losing weight and keeping it off than those who don't record their intake. A food journal helps you keep track of what you're eating and how many calories you're taking in

(continued on page 24)

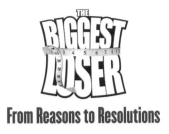

From Reasons to Resolutions

Like the cast members of *The Biggest Loser,* you too may have some deeply personal reasons for losing weight. But how strong is the resolve behind those reasons to actually lose weight and get in shape? To turn those reasons into heartfelt resolutions and achievable goals, answer the following questions.

Why do you want to lose weight? List the most important reasons you can think of—for example, to look better, have more energy, be able to play sports, be more self-confident, improve specific aspects of your health, and so forth.

_____

_____

_____

_____

_____

Next, take each of those reasons and reflect upon how your life will improve if you address them. For example: How will looking better benefit you? With more energy, what will you do that you're not doing now? How will playing sports enrich your life? Why do you want to be more confident, and how will it improve your life? What will your life be like in the absence of overweight-related health problems? How will you feel if you do all these things?

_____

_____

_____

_____

_____

_____

_____

_____

_____

Finally, set some weekly, doable goals for yourself to help you move forward in a positive manner. Depending on what you wrote above, ask yourself such questions as:

What can I do this week to improve my appearance?

_____

_____

_____

_____

What can I do this week that will increase my energy?

_____

_____

_____

_____

What sports, exercise, or other physical activity can I do this week to improve my fitness? When and how often will I do it?

_____

_____

_____

_____

What can I do this week to boost my self-confidence?

_____

_____

_____

_____

What actions will I take this week to improve my health?

_____

_____

_____

_____

each day. Further, it keeps you accountable, honest, and less susceptible to impulse eating during the day.

Be honest with what you write down. Jillian explained, "You need to track what you eat in detail. Not 'peanuts,' but how many peanuts? What time of day? And why are you eating just then? Writing it down makes you accountable and aware, and it helps you identify the mistakes you're making. Maybe your blood sugar is fluctuating through the day. Maybe you're skipping meals. Maybe you feel like you're not eating that much but, when you add it up, it comes to 2,500 calories a day."

As Jillian pointed out, a food journal can help you get to know your eating habits. Do you binge when eating your favorite foods? Do you eat when you're depressed or worried? Do you use food as a reward? Keeping track of your eating habits in a food journal may help you cut down on how much you eat, breaking the chains of behavior that lead to bingeing and emotional overeating.

A simple spiral-bound notebook makes a great food journal.

Weight Scale

To stay on track, it is important to weigh yourself at least weekly to detect changes in your weight when losing pounds. If you don't have one, you'll need a scale to weigh yourself.

Cast members on *The Biggest Loser* not only were weighed in pounds lost, they also had their body fat measured. The measurement of total body fat is considered to be a more useful piece of information than your weight, which is simply the grand total of your muscle, fat, bones, and other bodily tissue.

On the show, body-fat percentages were measured by underwater weighing, considered the gold standard of body-fat testing. The contestants were dunked in a tank, and their weight under water was used to calculate their body density. The information gained from this test is used to make calculations about body fat and lean muscle. Although very precise, this method is less accessible to the public.

If you want to know your body-fat percentage, along with your weight, you can purchase a home scale called a bioelectrical impedance scale, which analyzes body fat as a standard feature. This scale operates by measuring a signal that travels through your lower body, from one foot to the other. A faster signal means you have more muscle on your body. That's because water conducts electricity, and muscle is about 70 percent water; fat contains little water, so it "impedes" the signal. A range of 18 to 25 percent is generally considered healthy for women; for men, a healthy range is 10 to 18 percent.

Mantras for Motivation

When you're trying to lose weight, sometimes negative voices in your mind can trip you up. You might put too much pressure on yourself to succeed; then when you miss the mark, you beat yourself up over it. When you tried on a bathing suit, you felt unattractive and worthless. Evaluating yourself so harshly like that does nothing but make you want to throw in the towel and head for the doughnut shop. Or you tell yourself "I must get thin"—a mind-set that creates a sort of desperation in your outlook. Maybe you've told yourself that you will fail—again. Or when getting ready to work out, you say, "This is going to be hard," "I don't have any energy," "I don't have enough time"—all internal messages that cause your body to react with anxiety and stress. That kind of thinking immobilizes you and renders you hopeless. If you keep on thinking like this, you'll never change, since all of these attitudes interfere with weight-loss success.

That's why in season two, contestants were introduced to "mantras," positive affirmations to get them over these head-trip hurdles. These are invaluable for staying on course, nutritionally and with your exercise program.

Some examples of mantras appear in color on this page. By repeating mantras like these, you keep your attention centered and focused on what you need to do. What's more, you silence the negativity that goes on in your head. The effect is to create a new mental pattern of focusing on the positive, staying in the present, and not worrying about the future. Using mantras is like any other skill—the more you practice them, the more they'll eventually become part of your positive thought process.

• • •

Now that you've got your tools in front of you, you're ready to start "fixing" your weight. The first job: your diet. You'll be introduced to an eating plan that is neither drastic nor unhealthy, but one that's easy to incorporate into your life because it's designed for real life. Years down the road, when you're slim, trim, and fit, you'll be glad you found this plan. It's just what you need to transform your body, your health, and your life.

KEEP ON KEEPING ON

You Can Do It

I'm Prepared for Today's Workout

I Have a Strong, Healthy Body

I Can Do This

I LOOK GREAT

Just One More Mile

I Feel Great

ONE DAY AT A TIME

Fit Feels Good

I'm Beautiful

3 The Biggest Loser Diet:
EAT TO LOSE

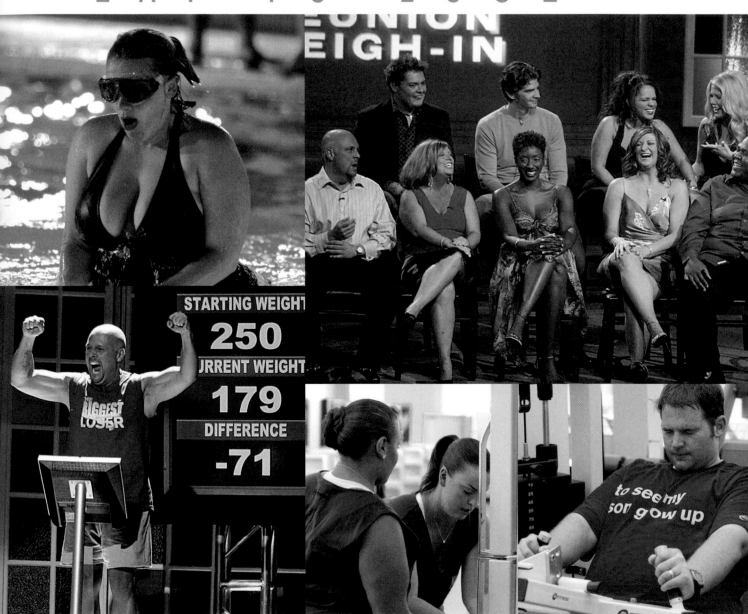

REUNION
WEIGH-IN

STARTING WEIGHT
250
CURRENT WEIGHT
179
DIFFERENCE
-71

to see my
son gow up

We know that when you flipped to this chapter, the first questions on your mind were: Will this diet work? What makes it different from every other diet I've tried?

Your questions are perfectly legit, and we want to answer them right away. And we're going to do that by having some of the Biggest Losers tell you why it works for them, both while they lose weight and more important, while they keep it off.

Kelly MacFarland, who lost 63 pounds (down from 223 pounds), says: "I'm a recovered fat girl, so I've tried every fad diet that's out there. They work for a while, but it's not a lifestyle. This diet is a lifestyle. It gives me consistency, flexibility, and variety in my eating so that when the unexpected event, birthday, or dinner out with friends happens, it's easy to follow and stay with."

Jen Kersey has lost 64 pounds so far on the diet since she weighed in at 267 pounds at the ranch. What she likes about the diet is the wide range of foods you get to eat. "I've learned how to make low-fat spaghetti and meatballs, low-fat Alfredo sauce, veggie fajitas, turkey chili, and all sorts of healthy, delicious foods. With this diet, there's a whole new world of eating out there."

Before appearing on *The Biggest Loser,* David Fioravanti was tipping the scales at well over 250 pounds; today he weighs in at a toned 183. "For me, this diet is 90 percent of losing weight; exercise is the other 10 percent," he says. "It's good clean eating, calorie-watching, with multiple meals spread out over the day. The foods are not only really tasty, but also good for you. It's a fun diet and it's a lifestyle."

Dana DeSilvio puts it very succinctly: "There are healthy diets, and there are unhealthy diets. This is a healthy one you can stick to. It doesn't even feel like a diet anymore; it's just my way of living." Dana started the show weighing in at 175 pounds and has now dieted and exercised down to 147. She's planning to enter a bathing suit competition for Planet Beach (a tanning company) very soon.

"This diet supplied the missing piece for me," said Pete Thomas, who has been losing weight steadily each week, thanks

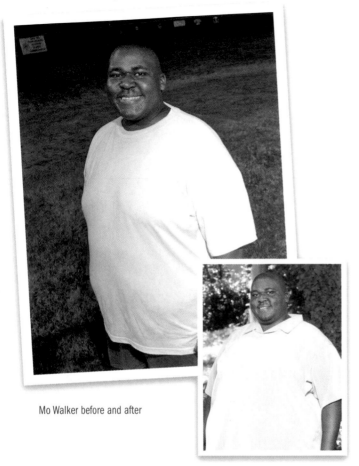

Mo Walker before and after

just about every diet that's out there. My weight was really at the point of where it was a do-or-die situation," he says. "About 2 weeks before the show started, I went to a doctor's appointment, and he told me that if I didn't do something about my weight, I would be dead in 5 years. Hearing that piece of bad news really motivated me to do something."

Mo started reducing his calories, carbs, and fat, watching his sodium level, and drinking at least 72 ounces of water daily. He pared off 80 pounds on the diet and also exercised to help shed weight.

So you see: Losing weight doesn't have to be something really radical, grueling, or punishing. It can be easy. It can be fun. And it can be permanent.

Introduction to the Biggest Loser Diet

The Biggest Loser diet is a calorie-controlled, carbohydrate-modified, fat-reduced diet geared to help you burn pound after pound of pure fat—and do so without deprivation or loss of energy. What's more, the diet is high in lean protein. Protein has a hunger-controlling effect on the body—which is why higher-protein diets are so effective for weight loss and fat burning.

While on this diet, you have the freedom to eat a wide variety of foods, as long as you stick to mostly whole, natural foods. "Whole foods" are those that have not been modified from their natural state or have been modified only a little bit, for example, through cooking. Foods that have been substantially modified are classified as processed

to the diet and a vigorous exercise program. "The piece I learned here is calories in, calories out. It's been broken down to basic math, and that has been very helpful. I've learned to watch my caloric intake and keep it around 1,500 to 1,800 calories a day, while working off as many more calories as I can. The weight is coming off." After the first 56 days of following the diet and exercising, Pete lost an amazing 76 pounds, down from his starting weight of 401.

Mo Walker weighed 436 pounds when he joined the show. "That was the heaviest that I've ever been. I had tried foods. Blueberries are a whole food. Blueberry toaster pastries are not.

Why is this important?

When you choose foods that are closer to their natural source, particularly fruits, vegetables, and whole grains, your body processes and uses them much more efficiently to build health. Whole foods are higher in fiber, which aids in weight loss, both because it is filling and because it helps reduce the number of calories that your body absorbs after a meal. Further, whole foods are much less fattening than processed foods because they do not contain added sugar or other sweeteners. Nor do they contain added fats or oils.

Bottom line: This diet will give you a healthy new way of eating that will help you manage your weight, and feel satisfied while you're doing it.

(For definitions of important nutrients, see "Diet Dictionary" on page 44.)

Calories—They're Back!

So far, we haven't said too much about the "C" word—calories, which is basically the measurement of how much energy a food gives you after you eat it. That energy is used by your body to fuel physical activity, as well as all metabolic processes, from maintaining your heartbeat and growing hair to healing a broken bone and building lean muscle. Only four components of food supply calories: protein and carbohydrates (4 calories per gram), alcohol (7 calories per gram), and fat (9 calories per gram). Vitamins, minerals, phytochemicals, fiber, and water do not supply calories.

No matter what you've heard, calories really do count in your diet, and they count big time. If you don't eat fewer calories than you burn off, you won't lose weight. Period. Game over. End of story.

Yes, there's a lot of controversy out there about the kind of diet you should eat for weight loss—low-carb, low-fat, or low-calorie. One of the reasons low-carb and low-fat diets work is that cutting carbs and cutting fat ultimately cuts calories. Remember, a calorie deficit is needed for weight loss, and these diets work to reduce calories, pure and simple. The Biggest Loser diet gives you the exact calorie deficit you require for your individual needs but without making you feel deprived of food.

How Many Calories Do You Need?

In calculating calories for weight loss, some formulas can get pretty elaborate, requiring you to do a lot of math. Not ours. We have a simple formula for you, put together by *The*

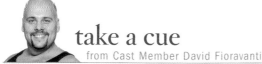

take a cue
from Cast Member David Fioravanti

The most important thing is to be consistent. There is nothing worse than saying, "I didn't eat all day, so I'll have a pizza." Or "I worked out so hard today that I'm going to chow down on Chinese food." No! You should say, "I worked out really hard today, so I'm going to eat really well to get the most out of my workout."

Biggest Loser doctors and nutritionists. Grab your calculator; here's the arithmetic:

Your present weight x 7 = Your daily caloric needs for weight loss

If you don't like doing math, the chart below gives you an idea of how many calories you need, depending on your current weight.

Your calorie count should *never* be static; in fact, it's a moving target. As you lose weight on this plan—and you will—you'll need to readjust your daily calories downward in order to keep losing weight at a good pace and break through plateaus, should your weight loss ever seem stalled.

If you weigh more than 300 pounds, start by eating 2,100 calories a day. If you weigh less than 150 pounds, plan to eat around 1,050 calories a day.

Current Weight	Daily Caloric Needs for Weight Loss
150	1,050
160	1,120
170	1,190
180	1,260
190	1,330
200	1,400
210	1,470
220	1,540
230	1,610
240	1,680
250	1,750
260	1,820
270	1,890
280	1,960
290	2,030
300	2,100

Make sure you keep something in mind: Everyone is different, and we all burn different amounts of calories at different rates. So if you and a partner, friend, or buddy follow this diet, one of you might lose weight at a different rate, faster or slower, than the other from week to week. Just like the contestants on *The Biggest Loser,* you may have huge losses one week, yet stay the same or even go up a pound the next. Ryan Benson, who ended up winning season one, dropped 19 pounds the first week, yet in week two, he lost 3 pounds—a more normal drop in weight for most dieters.

Losing a lot of weight is not always stacked in favor of men, either. In season two, when we pitted the men against the women, the women lost more weight than the men did the first week. So gals: Be encouraged and be empowered. There *is* equal opportunity when it comes to weight loss.

For both sexes, losing weight is a process of adaptation and equalizing. It's never a straight path to your goal. There will be plateaus, but there will also be huge windfalls. This is perfectly normal. Weight loss is always faster in the beginning because that's when you have more to lose, but it can slow down as you get closer to your goal.

The 4-3-2-1 Biggest Loser Pyramid

By now, you've probably seen or heard of the government's Food Guide Pyramid. Recently revised, it sets out a specified number of servings a day from various food groups. Using a pyramid is a great visual tool to help people remember what to eat each day, so that's why the medical and nutritional team at *The Biggest Loser* put together its own

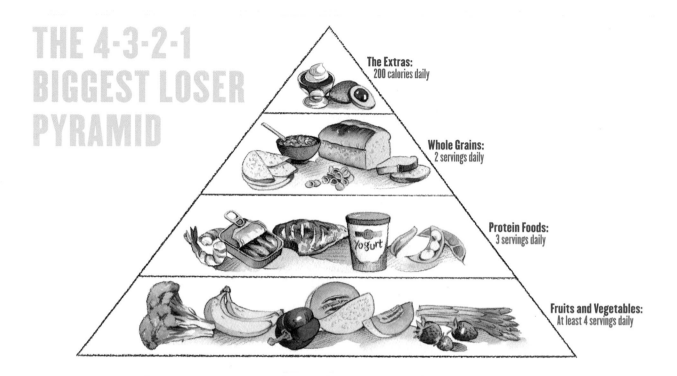

THE 4-3-2-1 BIGGEST LOSER PYRAMID

The Extras:
200 calories daily

Whole Grains:
2 servings daily

Protein Foods:
3 servings daily

Fruits and Vegetables:
At least 4 servings daily

version of the Food Guide Pyramid. We call it the 4-3-2-1 Biggest Loser Pyramid.

Illustrated above, our pyramid has fruits and vegetables at its base, protein foods on the second tier, and whole grains on the third tier. The small section at the tip gives you a 200-calorie budget for any food not included on the lower three tiers.

The food groups represented on our pyramid provide most of the nutrients you need daily. You should try to center your diet around the foods at the base of the pyramid and eat fewer servings from the foods toward the top of the pyramid.

Let's take a more detailed look at exactly what you

should be eating, and how much, in order to lose weight on the Biggest Loser diet.

The Biggest Loser Diet
1. Fruits and Vegetables: 4 Servings Daily, Minimum

At least half of your servings should be from vegetables; the other half from fruits. Don't have more fruit servings than vegetable servings.

Fruit Serving Size: 1 cup, 1 medium piece, or 8 ounces

Choose These to Lose: Apple, apricot, banana, blackberries, blueberries, cherries, cranberries, grapefruit, grapes, guava, kiwifruit, mango, melon (all varieties), nectarine, orange, papaya, peach, pear, persimmons, pineapple, plantain, plum, pomegranate, raspberries, rhubarb, strawberries, tangerine, and watermelon

Vegetable Serving Size: 1 cup or 8 ounces

Choose These to Lose: Artichoke, asparagus, bamboo shoots, beans (green, yellow), beet greens, beets, bell peppers, broccoli, brussels sprouts, cabbage, carrots, cauliflower, celery, collard greens, cucumbers, eggplant, kale, kohlrabi, leeks, lettuce (all varieties), mushrooms, mustard greens, okra, onions, palm hearts, parsley, peas, peppers (all varieties), pumpkin, radishes, shallots, spinach, sprouts, summer squash, sweet potatoes, Swiss chard, tomatillos, tomatoes, turnip greens, turnips, water chestnuts, watercress, winter squash, yams, and zucchini

Biggest Loser Pyramid Pointers

- Good news: You can eat more than four servings a day of most fruits and vegetables if you wish. At the base of our pyramid, fruits and vegetables supply the most nutrients in the form of vitamins, minerals, "phytochemicals" (protective plant chemicals), and fiber, relative to the low number of calories they contain. In other words, you get the most nutrient bang for your caloric buck from fruits and vegetables. The exception to this would be the starchier vegetables such as pumpkin, winter squash, sweet potatoes, and yams. These veggies are higher in calories and carbs, so you want to eat just a few servings a week.
- Fresh fruits and vegetables are always best, but when you can't get them that way, feel free to choose frozen or canned, as long as they are not packed with sugar or in syrup. Cooking and canning destroy some nutrients; however, the best food companies can their foods right after they're harvested, when they're the most fresh anyway.
- Eat a vegetable salad most days of the week.
- Cook your vegetables for the shortest amount of time possible in order to preserve nutrients.
- Keep a container of cut-up vegetables like broccoli and red or green peppers in your refrigerator for easy snacking.
- One vegetable to avoid while you're losing weight is white potatoes. Though nutritious, white potatoes send your blood sugar soaring. When it drops, you'll get hungry and be tempted to overeat at your next meal.
- Try a new fruit or vegetable every week to build some variety into your diet.
- Through the week, choose fruits and vegetables from

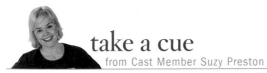

take a cue
from Cast Member Suzy Preston

I'm in my car all day, so I bring a bag of lettuce mixed with grilled chicken and a serving of salad dressing. When it's time for lunch, I just shake everything up and eat it out of the bag. This is a very convenient way to pack a nutritious lunch.

the six key color groups: red, orange, yellow, light green, dark green, and purple. This is a great way to make sure you're getting a variety of nutrients in your diet.

- Try to eat at least one fruit and one vegetable raw each day.
- Avoid dried fruits, including raisins, craisins, dried cherries, and dried blueberries. Dried fruits are often treated with additives, and they are overly concentrated in calories and fruit sugar, which can play havoc with your blood sugar. Further, they're not as filling as raw fruits, so they do little to help curb hunger. Consider this: Two tablespoons of raisins have as many calories as a whole cupful of grapes. Wouldn't you much rather eat a whole cup of grapes than a little bit of raisins?
- Choose whole fruits over fruit juices. Fruit juice contains no fiber and therefore does little to help you control your appetite or make you feel full. What's more, fruit juice is a concentrated source of fruit sugar and is thus liable to send your blood sugar soaring, followed by a decline. These ups and downs can lead to food cravings.

2. Protein Foods: 3 Servings Daily

The Biggest Loser Pyramid recommends three 8-ounce or 1-cup portions of protein foods each day, regardless of your daily caloric limit or target. For flexibility, you can choose from three different types of protein: animal protein, vegetarian protein, and low-fat dairy protein. You can divide your protein up into any size portion you want through the day. For example, you can have half a portion at breakfast, lunch, and dinner and for snacks, as long as you fulfill your protein allotment for the day. Protein is best eaten in smaller quantities anyway, so your body can use it throughout the day. So make sure you have some protein at each meal. Here is a closer look at your many protein choices.

Adding Protein to Your Daily Menu

Protein foods vary widely in calories, so making the right protein choice for your caloric needs is important. Below are guidelines that will let you select protein foods consistent with your caloric target.

Lower calorie targets (1,050 to 1,399 calories). If you're in this range, you'll need to select low-fat dairy as a protein source most frequently because it is low in calories and because the calcium in dairy foods is especially important for bone health in people with the lower caloric needs. The Biggest Loser diet thus recommends two servings of low-fat dairy proteins daily. Your third serving should come from animal protein, vegetarian protein, or a combination of the two.

Midrange calorie targets (1,400 to 1,799 calories). If you're aiming for a caloric intake in the midrange (1,400 to 1,800 calories), the Biggest Loser diet recommends one or two servings of low-fat dairy daily. Your remaining protein servings should come from animal protein, vegetarian protein, or a combination of the two.

Higher calorie targets (1,800 to 2,100 calories). Aim for at least 1 serving of low-fat dairy each day. Protein sources other than dairy should be used to reach your allotment of three protein servings daily.

Many of you will want to select one serving of fish, poultry, or meat on a daily basis, while others with a higher caloric target might choose to have an additional half or full serving of these higher-calorie protein foods on some days. Protein sources such as egg whites, beans, and soy foods are excellent daily protein choices for everyone, regardless of your caloric goals.

Animal Protein Serving Size: 1 cup or 8 ounces

Choose These to Lose: Any type of beef, pork, or veal labeled as 95 percent lean; white meat chicken; white meat turkey; egg whites; fish (any type); and shellfish (any type). Try to choose fish that is rich in heart-protective fats called omega-3 fatty acids. These fish include salmon, sardines (water-packed), herring, mackerel, trout, and tuna.

Vegetarian Protein Serving Size: 1 cup or 8 ounces

Choose These to Lose: Beans and legumes (black beans, broad beans, chickpeas, edamame, great Northern beans, kidney beans, lentils, lima beans, navy beans, pinto beans, split peas, white beans, and so forth); miso; soybeans, soy bacon, soy or veggie burgers, soy hot dogs, and other natural (meaning not the powders or pills) soy products; tempeh; and tofu

Low-Fat Dairy Serving Size: 1 cup or 8 ounces

Choose These to Lose: Buttermilk, low-fat milk (1 percent), skim or fat-free milk, soy milk, yogurt (plain), yogurt (no sugar added, fruit flavored), and reduced-fat cottage cheese

Biggest Loser Pyramid Pointers

- Ideally, try to choose a variety of proteins each day, as noted above in order to meet your calorie target. For example, with breakfast, you might have a cup of yogurt; with lunch, a cup of kidney beans as part of a vegetarian chili; as part of a snack, ½ cup of cottage cheese and with dinner, 4 ounces of grilled salmon.

- Especially in their menopausal years, women require ample calcium, available from low-fat dairy proteins. For that reason, women at this age may want to select two servings of protein from the low-fat dairy category, and the other serving from either animal proteins or vegetarian protein.

- For variety, consider soy foods such as soy hot dogs, soy sausage, and even soy pastrami because they contain no saturated fat. You can find them at your local natural food store and in many mainstream grocery stores.

- Before cooking poultry, remove the skin. This greatly reduces the fat and calorie content.

- Fish is an excellent source of low-calorie protein, heart-healthy omega-3 fatty acids, vitamin E, and selenium. Farm-raised seafood tends to be high in toxins called PCBs and other chemicals, although recent advance-

take a cue
from Cast Member Andrea ("Drea") Baptiste

If you crave chocolate, go buy some fat-free, sugar-free chocolate pudding, sprinkle a little cocoa powder in it to get that real chocolate taste, and you've got a great chocolate treat. When I feel like having some ice cream, I whip some cottage cheese to a creamy consistency, put a little almond extract or some crushed almonds in it for flavoring, put it in the freezer, and it becomes like frozen yogurt.

ments in fish farming have led to reduced levels of these toxins. If you are concerned about this issue, you may want to purchase wild fish. It is usually more expensive, however.

- Consider replacing conventionally raised meat or poultry with free-range or grass-fed meat or poultry. These foods contain more healthy fats and less saturated fat than conventionally raised meats and are free of antibiotics and growth hormone.
- Go easy on red meat. Limit your servings to twice a week, since red meat tends to be high in saturated fat.
- Avoid processed meats, such as bologna, hot dogs, salami, and so forth. Not only are they generally high in fat, these foods contain sodium nitrites, which react with foods in your stomach to form highly carcinogenic (potentially cancer-causing) compounds.

3. Whole Grains: 2 Servings Daily

Bread Serving Size: 2 slices bread, preferably "light," 1 whole-grain bun or roll, 2 light Wasa flatbreads, 1 whole-wheat flour tortilla

Choose These to Lose: Whole grain bread, high-fiber bread (choose brands with around 45 calories per slice); Ezekiel bread; Wasa bread; whole wheat buns, whole wheat pitas, whole wheat tortillas, and whole wheat dinner rolls

Whole Grain Serving Size: 1 cup cooked

Choose These to Lose: Barley, brown rice, bulgur, corn grits, couscous, cream of rice, cream of wheat, millet, oat bran, quinoa, rolled oats, whole wheat cereal, whole wheat pasta, and wild rice

Biggest Loser Pyramid Pointers

- For maximum nutrition, always lean toward the most nutritious grains—those that have undergone the least processing, such as those listed above. Brown rice, for example, is higher in vitamins and fiber than white rice. That's because white rice has been stripped of its husk, germ, and bran layers during processing. Similarly, rolled oats are more nutritious than instant oats. When grains are put through the process of refinement, the important nutrients are taken out. All that's usually left is the starchy interior, which is loaded with carbohydrates and not much else.
- To purchase the most nutritious bread products, read labels. Make sure the first ingredient listed is "whole" wheat or "whole grain." If "wheat flour" is the first ingredient, this doesn't mean whole wheat. It usually means enriched flour with some whole wheat added.
- Choose breads with 2 or more grams of fiber per serving.

 take a cue
from Cast Member Dana DeSilvio

Take a picture of yourself at your worst—with your belly hanging out or a spare tire around your waist. Post that picture on your refrigerator and keep telling yourself you don't want to look like that.

- Again, watch out for the term "enriched" on the label when buying bread or pasta. It's usually a sign that a food is made with processed white flour, meaning that it's low in fiber. Usually, the nutrients have been stripped and then replaced synthetically.
- Avoid most packaged ready-to-eat breakfast cereals. These tend to be highly processed and loaded with added sugar. Some exceptions are low-carb cereals (a favorite among cast members) and high-fiber cereals such as Kashi Go Lean, Fiber One, and All-Bran. Packaged cereals containing 5 grams of fiber or more per serving are generally considered to be high-fiber cereals.

  Another factor to consider when choosing a breakfast cereal is its sugar content. Although all cereals will naturally have some sugar in them, you want to avoid cereals that have a great deal of added sugar. Read the label for sugar content. A good rule of thumb that's easy to remember is to choose packaged cereals with less than 5 grams of sugars and at least 5 grams of fiber per serving.

4. The Extras: Your 200-Calorie Budget

You are allotted 200 extra calories a day in addition to what you eat from the foods above. The goal here is to spend your budget on healthy choices and not squander it on nutritionally bankrupt foods such as candy or sweets. Sensible, healthy choices include the following foods and condiments:

Fats, Oils, and Spreads

- Good fats such as olive oil, canola oil, flaxseed oil, or walnut oil
- Reduced-fat and fat-free salad dressings and mayonnaise
- Reduced-fat peanut butter and nut butters

Sugar-Free Desserts and Sweets

- Sugar-free, fat-free puddings and gelatins
- Reduced-calorie jams, jellies, and syrups
- Sugar-free popsicles and fudgsicles
- Sugar-free, fat-free whipped topping

Reduced-Fat Foods

- Reduced-fat or fat-free cheeses
- Fat-free sour cream

Condiments and Sauces

- Low-calorie barbecue sauce
- Reduced-sodium broths or bouillons

take a cue
from Cast Member Lizzeth Davalos

Who says you have to give up pizza? Make your own healthy version like I do. Spread some pizza sauce over a piece of pita bread. Top with your favorite pizza veggies, herbs, and some shredded low-fat cheese. Bake at 350°F until the cheese is bubbly and the pizza is hot, then enjoy!

- Low-calorie catsup
- Chili sauce
- Cocktail sauce
- Horseradish
- Mustard
- Picante sauce
- Salsa
- Lite soy sauce
- Steak sauce
- Tabasco sauce
- Tomato paste
- Tomato sauce
- Worcestershire sauce

Other

- Avocado
- Nuts and seeds
- Olives
- Pickles (unsweetened varieties)

Biggest Loser Pyramid Pointers

- Avoid animal fats (found in egg yolks, meat products, and full-fat dairy products) and trans fats (found in margarine and processed foods that feature "hydrogenated oil" on the ingredients list). Both kinds of fat can damage your cell membranes and interfere with your body's ability to use good fats that protect you against disease.
- Reduced-fat, sugar-free, fat-free, and low-carb products should be used sparingly in your diet. Your meals should be made up mostly of whole foods, with less emphasis on "diet-food" substitutes.
- Be careful with nuts and seeds. They pack a big caloric punch, and because they usually don't come packaged in single servings, it's far too easy to overindulge in them.
- If you're someone who likes to pour on the catsup, barbecue sauce, or salad dressings, make sure you use the low-calorie versions of your favorite condiments. Their carbs and calories have usually been reduced by replacing sugar, corn syrup, and other sweeteners with sugar substitutes. Switching to the low-calorie versions can save you a few calories.
- Feel free to uses spices and herbs to flavor your meals. For an added health kick, try antioxidant-rich choices like cumin, dill, garlic, ginger, lavender, mint, onions, oregano, parsley, rosemary, saffron, sage, thyme, and turmeric.
- Certain condiments such as soy sauce can be high in sodium, contributing to water retention. If sodium appears high on the list of ingredients, you may want to avoid that particular condiment or see if it comes in a low-salt or salt-free version. Unless you have high blood pressure, sodium isn't a big deal, but it will make you hold water temporarily. Water retention can make you look and feel fat and may hinder metabolism.

When to Adjust Your Calories

As you bid farewell to those pounds and inches, your calorie requirement will drop. You see, for every 1 pound of fat you lose, you decrease the number of calories you expend each day by about 10. That's roughly the number of calories that were required to keep that fat at body temperature, move it around, and support its metabolic needs. So when you shed 10 pounds of fat, you will be burning up about 100 fewer calories each day than you did when you weighed more. If you want to keep losing weight, you either have to eat fewer calories, exercise more, or do both. Unless you readjust your calories or your exercise, you'll reach equilibrium, or you may even start to gain weight. And that's not an option!

When it's time for you to reduce your calories, there are four easy, near-automatic ways to do so.

1. Cut your calories from your optional 200-calorie budget.
2. Replace your whole grain servings with vegetables.
3. Choose lower-calorie protein foods such as low-fat dairy, egg whites, and soy.
4. Reduce your fruit servings in favor of more vegetables.

Just don't get discouraged! It's highly unlikely that your weight will climb on this plan because the Biggest Loser diet keeps your calories, carbs, and fat in check.

Artificial Sweeteners

You may use artificial sweeteners in moderation, if you wish. Artificial sweeteners may help some people better manage their weight. Because they are many times sweeter than sugar, it takes much less of them to create the same sweetness, but with far fewer calories. Some people experience headaches when they use artificial sweeteners, so you'll have to choose one that agrees with you.

What to Drink

When you're on a losing-weight streak, the best drink of choice is water—and plenty of it. Recent studies show that water may play a role in the regulation of your metabolism—your body's calorie-burning engine. For one thing, if you become dehydrated, your metabolism tends to slow down, meaning that you won't burn as many calories as normal while at rest. In addition, ample water may reduce appetite and control food intake by making you feel full, and it dilutes sodium levels in the body, making it the best remedy for fluid retention.

If you're eating more protein and fiber and exercising more, as this diet and exercise program recommends, you'll

take a cue
from Cast Member Kelly MacFarland

If you're feeling hungry, make a "Protein Scramble." Sauté some egg substitute with some reduced-fat cheese, tomato, spinach, broccoli, or whatever veggie you have on hand. This snack really hits the spot.

need more water than normal. Aim for six to eight 1-cup servings of water or more a day.

If you can, drink your water ice cold. Your body needs to heat up this water in order to use it properly. Metabolically, heating up water takes energy. In other words, it burns up calories. In fact, you can automatically burn up an extra 50 to 100 calories a day by drinking just 4 to 8 cups of ice cold water.

Drinking water doesn't have to be boring, either. Try flavoring a pitcher of plain water with herbs like mint or basil or slices of citrus fruits or cucumber.

Other allowable beverages you may drink *in moderation* and *in addition to your water* are:

- No-calorie flavored water
- Coffee or tea, caffeinated or decaffeinated
- Diet sodas (limit to one or two a day)
- Herbal teas

What about Alcoholic Beverages?

While you're following the Biggest Loser diet, alcohol isn't necessarily off-limits because you can build it into your daily calorie count. However, here are some points to consider carefully prior to imbibing: Alcoholic beverages supply calories (usually in the form of sugar) but few nutrients. A 12-ounce regular beer contains about 150 calories, a 5-ounce glass of wine about 100 calories, and 1.5 ounces of 80 proof distilled spirits about 100 calories. Drinking alcohol may also interfere with your body's ability to burn fat. Another benefit of abstaining: Drinking lowers your inhibitions and stimulates your appetite, making you more likely to splurge on poor food choices. While you can certainly enjoy alcohol every now and then, be careful because it could interfere with steady weight loss.

Meal Timing

While following the Biggest Loser diet, you'll eat four to six planned meals each day, including three main meals (breakfast, lunch, and dinner) and one to three snacks. There is enormous wisdom in doing so. Frequent eating:

- Helps regulate your appetite and tames carb and sugar cravings
- Keeps you from feeling deprived
- Helps control blood sugar and insulin levels (insulin is a fat-forming hormone)
- Leads to lower body fat

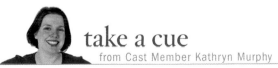

take a cue
from Cast Member Kathryn Murphy

When I'm craving something sweet, I grab a diet root beer. It cuts the need for sweetness.

- Keeps you energized for exercise and activity
- Reduces stress hormones in the body that can contribute to fat accumulation
- Establishes a regular pattern of eating that helps counter impulse eating

"The most important part of this diet to me was the eating every 3 hours," says *The Biggest Loser* cast member Kelly MacFarland. "I had never done that before. Eating a lot of food broke me out of the 'you have to eat like a bird' mold of losing weight."

Ryan Benson adds, "When I was fat, I used to eat two gigantic meals a day—which were really unhealthy. Now I have a sensible breakfast, a snack before lunch, two chicken breasts and a big salad for lunch, and then another snack of fruit in the afternoon. For dinner, I'll have a couple of turkey burgers and another large salad. I eat more times throughout the day, and this helps me stay where I am."

How to Structure Your Meals

Okay, now that you understand the basics of the Biggest Loser diet, let's talk about how to put your meals together. What follows is a template to help you create and structure your own meals. You don't have to follow this template exactly. Flexible and adaptable to your needs and tastes, it simply gives you a blueprint for planning your meals and arranging all your servings throughout the course of a day. For

example, you don't have to have fruit at breakfast; you might save it for a snack or another meal later. You'll also find sample 1-week menus for 1,200, 1,500, and 1,800-calorie diets in the appendix. These can be enormously helpful because they take all the guesswork out of meal planning and are a breeze to follow.

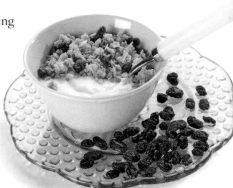

Breakfast

½ protein serving
1 whole grain serving
1 fruit serving

Snack

½ protein serving
1 fruit serving

Lunch

1 protein serving
½ whole grain
1 vegetable serving

Snack

½ protein serving
1 fruit serving

Dinner

½ protein serving
½ whole grain serving
2 vegetable servings

Extra

200 calories from additional foods, healthy fats, and condiments

If you filled in the template with allowable foods from the Biggest Loser diet food lists above, your menu for 1 day might look something like this.

Breakfast

½ cup egg whites, scrambled, with 1 teaspoon basil, and *1 teaspoon grated reduced-fat Parmesan cheese

2 slices whole wheat toast

1 cup diced cantaloupe

Snack

1 cup fresh berries topped with ½ cup sugar-free fruit-flavored yogurt

Lunch

Southwestern Bulgur Salad, made with ½ cup cooked bulgur wheat, 4 ounces grilled chicken breast, 1 cup diced grilled vegetables (2 tablespoons onion, 6 tablespoons zucchini, ⅓ cup bell pepper, *2 tablespoons chopped avocado, and 1 teaspoon chopped cilantro), and *1½ tablespoons shredded low-fat cheese

Snack

½ cup reduced-fat cottage cheese

1 cup diced fresh pineapple

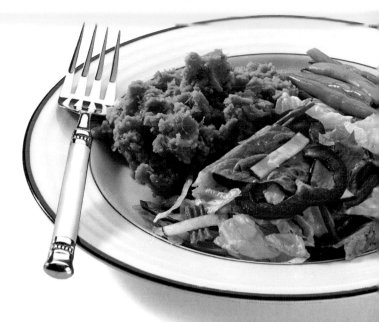

Dinner

4 ounces grilled salmon

½ cup brown rice

Tossed salad with 1½ cups mixed baby salad greens, ½ cup cherry tomatoes, and *1 tablespoon light Russian vinaigrette

*These foods would count as your extras in the 200-calorie budget.

Portion Power

With super-sized meals, Double Gulps, and king-size candy bars making their way onto the food scene, we're not surprised that it's so tough for people to win at weight loss. Huge portions are making *us* huge! Most people no longer have any idea of what constitutes a normal, healthy portion.

With the Biggest Loser diet, you'll learn what a healthy

portion really looks like by weighing and measuring your servings. If you don't have access to a scale and measuring cup, you can take portion control into your own hands— literally. One cup of whole grains, vegetables, or fruit, for example, is about the size of your clenched fist; one protein serving equals roughly the size of the palm of your hand.

But don't worry; you won't have to weigh and measure forever. In a few short weeks, you'll be able to eyeball the correct portions. And once your portions slim down, so will your body.

What to Avoid: Appetite-Stimulating Foods

If you're determined to be your own "Biggest Loser," but find yourself caving in to cravings, it could be that your food choices are partially sabotaging your efforts. Eating certain foods will make you so hungry that you'll feel hollow inside. We call these appetite-stimulating foods. These include any food that has been stripped of its fiber, such as white bread; foods that turn to sugar quickly in the body, such as white potatoes; and foods loaded with sugar, starch, and fat. Some examples include:

- White bread
- White pasta
- White potatoes
- Pastries
- Doughnuts
- Cookies

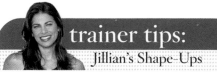

trainer tips:
Jillian's Shape-Ups

- When going to parties and picnics, avoid the booze. It will destroy your diet! If you must partake, allow yourself two drinks max and opt for the low-cal drinks like light beer or vodka and diet 7UP.
- Make your own healthy treats like popsicles. Try using Crystal Light or Diet Snapple to make your own popsicles—at less than 15 calories a popsicle. These beverages come in all kinds of flavors. The possibilities are endless! You can also make a yummy fruit salad with berries and fat-free Reddi Whip at only 5 calories a tablespoon.
- Don't let your vacation become a diet disaster! Just because you go on holiday does not give you license to completely abandon your diet. Make sure you bring healthy snacks on your trip. I always like to pack a couple of bags of raw almonds and a box of low-carb cereal just in case. And don't forget to exercise while you're away! By keeping those endorphins flowing, you'll not only burn calories but also maintain higher spirits and a high energy level.

- Cakes, pies, and other sugary baked goods
- Candy and candy bars
- Potato chips and other packaged and fried snacks

Why do these foods give you that irresistible urge to raid the fridge or pantry? It has to do with their composition. The more fiber that is removed from these foods, the harder and more rapidly they hit your bloodstream. The sugar and refined starch they contain causes your blood sugar to soar sky-high. In response to that sugar surge, your body churns out insulin—so much that it drives your blood sugar below where it was before you ate anything. When blood sugar is that low, you feel tired and hungry and in need of another quick pickup—often in the form of something sweet. These ups and downs, coupled with the wrong food choices, can wreak havoc on your attempts to manage your weight. When a food contains both fat and sugar, as many of the foods listed above do, it can be downright addictive since many of us crave the taste of fat and sugar.

The key, of course, is to avoid appetite-stimulating foods—and make a habit of reaching for natural, wholesome, high-fiber foods and snacks instead. These whole foods are digested more slowly, causing fewer spikes in your blood sugar. What's more, they tame your hunger, rather than drive it wild with those crazy blood sugar ups and downs. Trust us, before long, you'll lose your sugar/fat/starch tooth and be in better control of your cravings.

Read Labels

When it comes to losing weight, the more you know about the foods you're buying and eating, the better. The best way to educate yourself is to read the Nutrition Facts panel on the back of every manufactured food package.

Everything listed on the panel is important, but there are several items that you should really concern yourself with. "Translating Label Lingo" and the Diet Dictionary on page 44 will help you make sense of "labelese."

It is also important to pay attention to the list of ingredients. This portion of the label reveals hidden dangers, such as added sugars and trans fats. The more ingredients a food contains, the likelier the product is to be higher in calories. A good rule of thumb is to select foods with a shorter ingredient list. For example, plain yogurt contains only milk, live active cultures, and sometimes a thickening agent. Flavored yogurt has a much longer list of ingredients, including added sugars and starches, making it 100 calories higher per cup than plain.

Since being a contestant on *The Biggest Loser,* Dana DeSilvio has become an avid label reader. "Just recently, I was going to buy some canned peaches. I read the label, and it said 20 grams of sugar. I decided to buy a whole peach instead and cut it up myself—which gives me only naturally occurring sugar."

Watch out for the word "hydrogenated," too. It's a fancy name for trans fats, which are made by adding hydrogen to vegetable oil. These cheap, synthetic fats have been linked to an increased risk of heart disease and are frequently found in commercially baked goods and snacks.

Nutrition Facts		
Serving Size		
Servings Per Container		
Amount Per Serving		
Calories 0	Calories from Fat 0	
		% Daily Value*
Total Fat 0g		0%
Saturated Fat 0g		0%
Polyunsaturated Fat 0g		
Monounsaturated Fat 0g		
Cholesterol 0mg		0%
Sodium 0mg		0%
Total Carbohydrate 0g		0%
Dietary Fiber 0g		0%
Sugars 0g		
Protein 0g		
Vitamin A 0%	•	Vitamin C 0%
Calcium 0%	•	Iron 0%

* Percent Daily Values are based on a 2,000 calorie diet. Your daily values may be higher or lower depending on your calorie needs:

		Calories:	2,000	2,500
Total Fat	Less than		0g	0g
Sat Fat	Less than		0g	0g
Cholesterol	Less than		0mg	0mg
Sodium	Less than		0mg	0mg
Total Carbohydrate			0g	0g
Dietary Fiber			0g	0g

Carbohydrate. A macronutrient that comes from plants—vegetables, grains (like wheat, corn, oats, rice, and barley), beans, and fruits. Your body gets most of its energy from eating carbohydrates.

Protein. A macronutrient found in meat, fish, eggs, poultry, and dairy products, and in smaller amounts in beans, nuts, and whole grains. Protein is required to build and repair muscle, skin, hair, blood vessels, and other bodily tissues.

Saturated Fat. Fat that comes from animal foods (butter and lard, for example) and is generally solid at room tem-

Translating Label Lingo

Label	Definition
Serving Size	This refers to the standard amount of food suggested by the food manufacturer or by the U.S. Department of Agriculture. Knowing the serving size of various foods allows you to choose the one that's lower in calories. Watch out for foods that look as though they are a single serving package, but aren't. A good example is a 12-ounce bottle of fruit juice, which may actually contain 2 to 2½ servings.
Calories and Calories from Fat	For one day, less than 30 percent (30 in 100) of your calories should come from fat.
Total Fat	This value equals: grams of saturated fat + grams of polyunsaturated fat + grams of monounsaturated fat. A food that is low in fat contains no more than 3 grams of fat per serving.
Saturated Fat	Keep your saturated fat intake to less than one-third of your total fat intake. If you limit fat to 60 grams a day, for example, no more than 20 grams of it should come from saturated fat.
Cholesterol	Although cholesterol alone in food is not a big culprit in raising cholesterol levels in the body, you should still limit your cholesterol intake to 300 milligrams (mg) daily.
Sodium	Try to limit your sodium intake each day to less than 2,400 milligrams, especially if you already have high blood pressure, congestive heart failure, or fluid retention problems.
Total Carbohydrate	This value equals: grams of sugar + grams of fiber + grams of complex carbohydrate (usually not listed). If the amount of total carbohydrate is more than double the amount of sugars, that's a plus because there are more "good carbs" in the food.

perature. When saturated fat comes from tropical sources like coconuts, it's liquid at room temperature. Saturated fat, particularly from animal foods, is the artery-clogging type and is known to raise levels of unhealthy cholesterol in the body when eaten in excess.

Unsaturated Fats. These include polyunsaturated and monounsaturated fats. These are typically oils that come from plants like olives, corn, and soybeans, and from seafood. Eating these fats in the proper amounts tends to help you avoid clogged arteries.

Omega-3 Fat. A special type of fat in the diet that is considered essential, meaning that our bodies do not produce

Label	Definition
Sugars	Sugars include naturally present sugars, such as lactose in milk and fructose in fruits, and those added to foods, such as table sugar, corn syrup, honey, and dextrose. Added sugar in foods is detrimental to weight loss. That's because eating too much sugar stimulates your appetite, plus it drives insulin upward, causing calories to be converted into body fat. On food labels, sugar travels in disguise under names such as corn syrup, high-fructose corn syrup, fructose, maltose, molasses, fruit juice concentrate, brown sugar, invert sugar, corn sweetener, lactose, raw sugar, glucose, dextrose, table sugar, syrup, and honey.
Fiber	Anything above 2 or 3 grams is considered a good source of fiber, and "high-fiber foods" are those containing 5 or more grams of fiber per serving. The more fiber, the better. A good rule of thumb is to limit foods that have more than 7 grams of total carbohydrates per gram of fiber. Such foods are probably overly processed and fiber-poor. Example: If a food contains 3 grams of fiber, there should be no more than 21 grams of total carbohydrates. The higher in fiber a food is, the likelier it is to be lower in calories. Aim to get at least 25 grams of fiber each day. Among your best bets are legumes, like chickpeas, pinto beans, and lentils, which offer 5 to 7 fiber grams per half-cup serving. And don't forget fresh fruits and veggies: They'll give you 2 to 8 grams of fiber per 1-cup serving.
Protein	Generally speaking, anything above 9 grams of protein per serving means the food is a high-protein food.
Vitamins and Minerals	If the percentages are above 10, that's good; above 20, even better.
Percent Daily Values	This is general information explaining that the percentage numbers listed for nutrients are based on a 2,000 calorie diet. (Of course, a person's daily nutrient requirements may be higher or lower depending on caloric needs.)

it, and therefore, it is essential we include it in our diets. Omega-3 fats appear to decrease risk of many types of cancer and heart disease. Fatty fish such as salmon is a good source of these fats.

Trans Fats or Partially Hydrogenated Oils. These are man-made fats, created when vegetable oil is hardened to make margarine, for example. Used in many baked goods and junk foods, trans fats can clog your arteries when eaten in excess.

Cholesterol. A waxy substance made by your liver that is needed for good cellular health. It is also found in animal fat and can be harmful when we eat too much because it deposits in our arteries, blocking bloodflow.

Vitamins. Micronutrients that come from living things—plants and animals. Vitamins help your body use protein, carbohydrates, and fat.

Minerals. Chemical elements such as calcium, iron, and potassium, found in foods, that are necessary for life and for good health.

Fiber. The indigestible portion of plant foods that produces a feeling of fullness and helps maintain good digestive health.

Antioxidants. A nutrient that can counteract the damaging effects of oxygen in tissues. Examples are beta-carotene, vitamin C, and vitamin E.

Phytochemicals. Substances in plants that may possess health-protective benefits, even though unlike vitamins and minerals, they are not essential for life.

Macronutrient. These are substances your body needs in relatively large amounts. Carbohydrates, proteins, and fats are examples of macronutrients.

Micronutrient. These are substances your body needs in small amounts. Vitamins and minerals are examples of micronutrients.

The Biggest Loser Diet Recap

- Deal with hunger before it happens. Eat four to six meals a day, one about every 3 hours. You'll get a constant supply of the fuel and nutrients your body needs and avoid feeling overly hungry.
- Adjust your caloric intake as you lose weight.
- Choose healthy whole foods and lean proteins.
- Use the 4-3-2-1 Biggest Loser Pyramid to guide your food choices every day.
- Drink six to eight 8-ounce glasses of water a day.
- Watch your portion sizes. An 8-ounce serving is approximately the size of your hand; a 4-ounce serving is the size of your palm.
- Avoid appetite-stimulating foods.
- Read labels.

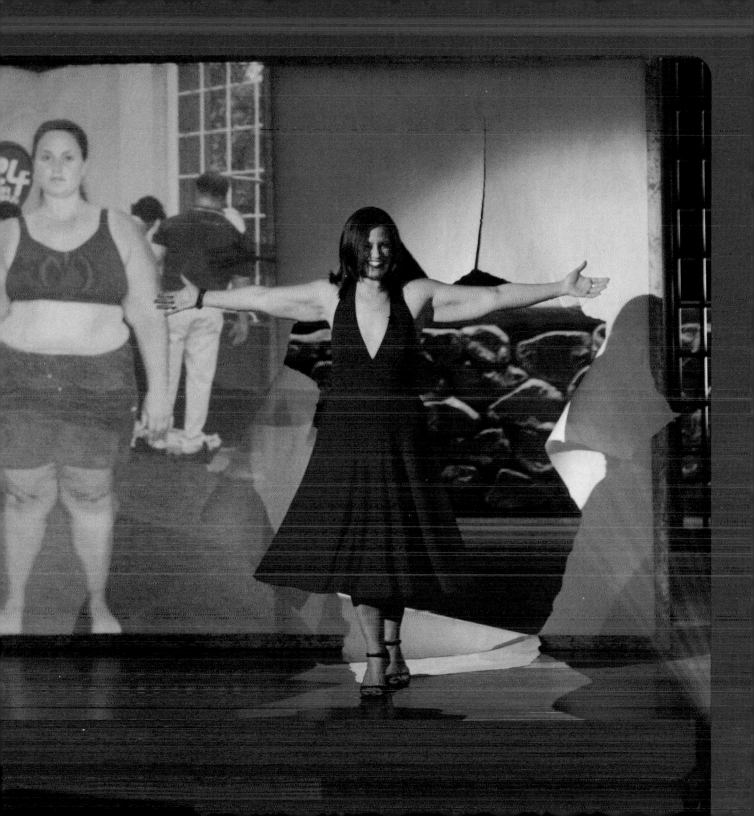

4 The Biggest Loser

EXERCISE PLAN

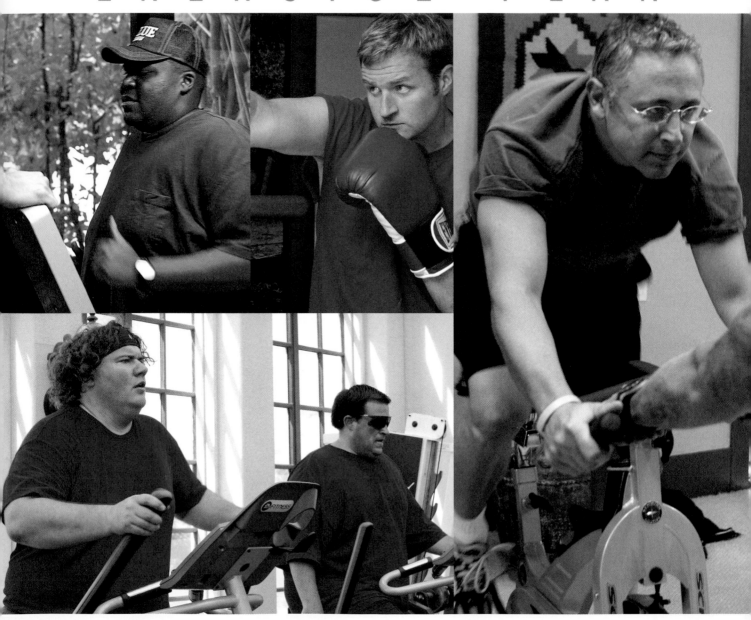

The key to becoming a big loser is mathematically very simple: Eat less, move more. We've just covered the "eat less" part of the equation; now it's time to talk about moving more. Remember, 1 pound of body fat equals 3,500 calories. By burning 250 to 500 calories a day through exercise, you could lose up to a whole pound a week (7 x 500 = 3,500), as long as you push yourself actively and don't go overboard on fattening foods.

To get you moving and losing, the Biggest Loser exercise plan will nuke calories and fat by keeping your metabolism and motivation charged up. At its core is a 12-week cardio workout that increases the intensity of your aerobic training for a fat-blasting boost. You'll alternate this routine with a circuit training routine that uses nine specific moves in a sequence, with only several seconds of rest between sets. This routine, which boosts your metabolism, will take you no longer than 30 minutes, just three times a week. When you're feeling stronger and more energetic, you'll gradually up your repetitions, sets, and poundages. Put it all together and you'll melt fat, get more toned, look more sculpted, and feel energized!

One thing that's important to understand about this exercise plan is that it does not require the 4 to 6 (or more) rigorous hours of exercising that *The Biggest Loser* cast members went through every day. Because the show was a competition to see who could lose the most weight, the goal was to burn up as many calories—and as much fat—as possible in a day. That way, each contestant could experience dramatic weight losses from week to week. In the real, everyday world, people require a more moderate program, but one with the same end point in mind: Burn off the pounds.

This plan is designed to do just that: Target, attack, and incinerate your body fat. You'll get significant results in a faster-than-normal amount of time. You won't waste your time on anything that does not take you straight to your goal of burning calories and fat and dropping pounds. Rest assured, this is a safe, healthy way to exercise and is not some sort of gimmicky quick-fix deal. After all, *The Biggest Loser* is about getting healthy and losing weight the good old-fashioned way—by diet and exercise. All that is asked of you is that you work hard for the next 12 weeks, at intensities that accommodate your improving level of fitness.

As you start out, you'll need to accept the fact that the first few days may not be fun. You've just got to push through. Your body is an amazing machine. After 2 weeks, the walk that used to have you sucking wind won't even tire you out. It took only that long for the cast on *The Biggest Loser* to discover they could do exercises they initially found impossible. By the end of the first 4 weeks, you'll see some pretty significant changes.

In the end, you will love the way your body looks and feels. You'll be a new person, inside and out. You will have transformed your body and your life and altered your mental and motivational makeup by challenging yourself to go farther than ever before.

Outside Shape Starts on the Inside

For the trainers on the show, one of the biggest challenges of *The Biggest Loser* was to help a group of people gain control of their lives—even after they had let themselves go. At the very beginning of the show, the trainers approached their teams from the inside out. They told the cast it wasn't just going to be about what to eat, what not to eat, and how to exercise. The cast had to start feeling great about their bodies—*before they got great bodies.* They had to get comfortable in their own skin, be accepting and loving of where they were, and not be so wrapped up in the finished product.

What they did with the cast—which is what you'll do right now—was to get them to focus on what they liked about themselves. We are all so quick to say what we hate—but what about those qualities we like? In the same way you taught yourself to be your worst critic, you can just as easily teach yourself to feel more positive again. Success begins when you stop being so hard on yourself and celebrate everything you have going for you.

Think about it: What do you like about yourself right now? Take out a piece of paper and make a list of all your likable qualities. Keep going until this list is as long as you can make it. You might include things like *I have sexy eyes, I have thick hair, I can make people laugh, I am a good cook, I'm creative, I'm trustworthy, I'm a good friend,* or *I'm intelligent.*

Keep adding to this list as you get in better shape. Stay focused on all these positives, always. It's this type of thinking that will help you develop self-acceptance and body confidence. You'll start feeling much more fired up

take a cue
from Cast Member Kelly MacFarland

If anyone has an excuse not to work out, it's me. I have a full-time job; plus, four or five times a week, I'm on the road as a stand-up comedian. Even so, I feel like exercise is important to making my life work. Exercise is the one thing I do not sacrifice. I work out 6 days a week for about an hour and a half. Twice a week, I pull a "double"—another 45 minutes to an hour at night, usually some light cardio. Exercise makes my lungs strong. It clears my head. It makes me perform better. I do work a lot, but I make sure I take time for me. Exercise equals "me-time," in other words. You'll be more successful if you start looking at it from that point of view. Once you get that mind-set, it's easy to stick with it.

and in absolute awe of your own abilities and strengths. You'll start to feel good about the process involved in losing weight and not just the outcome.

The people who will be most successful at losing weight and keeping it off are those who are open and willing to do whatever it takes to make a healthy change in their lifestyles. They have a commitment within themselves to fix what's broken and the openness to allow it to happen.

What about you? Are you that person?

We know you can do it. Now let's get moving!

Find Your Level

A big plus of the Biggest Loser exercise plan is that it accommodates all levels of fitness. Week by week, this progressive program advances with you, whether you're a beginner, an intermediate exerciser, or an advanced exerciser. Read through these descriptions and pick the one that most closely describes your current fitness status.

Beginner: You are just beginning an exercise program for the first time or for the first time in a long time. Good for you! Most people just think about exercising and never actually do anything about it. You will feel so much better for acting on your goals.

Intermediate Exerciser: You've already been exercising fairly consistently for 3 months at least three times per week. Congratulations! Did you know that less than 25 percent of us actually exercise frequently enough to experience any health benefits? You should be very proud that you take the time to take care of yourself. Our fat-burning program

will help take your fitness to the next level and give you a greater challenge.

Advanced Exerciser: You've been exercising on a regular basis, perhaps as many as five or six times a week, and for many months or maybe for many years. That means you're an advanced exerciser—a title that very few people in our society have achieved. You probably already know the benefits of regular physical activity because you experience them as a result of your consistent efforts. This program will vary what you've been doing in the past, plus give you an extra challenge, so that you remain as excited about it forever!

The Fat-Burning Cardio Workout

With exercise, you must strive to burn as much fat as possible and a substantial number of calories. That's where cardio comes in. It's really what lights the fat-burning furnaces. This cardio workout involves two types of exercise: *steady-state cardio* and *interval cardio.*

Steady state means that you walk, jog, run, bike, or use a cardio machine for a specified period of time (usually 30 to 60 minutes), and you work out at an even pace. You're probably most familiar with steady-state cardio, also called continuous training. If you've ever gone for a 30-minute walk, run, or jog, for example, you've done a steady-state cardio workout. It is a great way to get your heart rate in its fat-burning zone and keep it there for a certain period of time.

Interval cardio alternates high-intensity exercise periods with periods of slower-paced work. Interval cardio can help

(continued on page 54)

Exercise Routine for the Fat-Burning Cardio Workout

In the following exercise routine, we're using walking and jogging as examples. Rather than walk or jog, you may also do other forms of cardio, including stationary cycling, treadmill walking, elliptical exercising, stair-climbing, or even a combination of these.

Cardio Workout	Beginner	Intermediate	Advanced
Week 1	Steady-state cardio: 20–30 minutes of fast-paced walking, 3 times a week.	Steady-state cardio: 30–45 minutes of fast-paced walking, 4 times a week.	Steady-state cardio: 45–60 minutes of fast-paced walking or jogging, 5 or 6 times a week.
Week 2	Steady-state cardio: 30 minutes of fast-paced walking, 3 times a week.	Steady-state cardio: 45–60 minutes of fast-paced walking, 4 times a week.	Steady-state cardio: 60 minutes of fast-paced walking or jogging, 5 or 6 times a week.
Week 3	Steady-state cardio: 30–45 minutes of fast-paced walking, 3 times a week. Increase intensity by walking faster or at a higher incline, or increase your level on a cardio machine.	Steady-state cardio: 45–60 minutes of fast-paced walking, 4 times a week. Increase intensity by walking faster or at a higher incline, or increase your level on a cardio machine.	Steady-state cardio: 60 minutes of fast-paced walking or jogging, 5 or 6 times a week. Increase intensity by walking faster or at a higher incline, or increase your level on a cardio machine.
Week 4	Steady-state cardio: 45 minutes of fast-paced walking, 4 times a week. Continue to increase intensity by walking faster, jogging or running, or working at a higher incline, or increase your level on a cardio machine.	Steady-state cardio: 60 minutes of fast-paced walking, 5 times a week. Continue to increase intensity by walking faster, jogging or running, or working at a higher incline, or increase your level on a cardio machine.	Steady-state cardio: 60 minutes of fast-paced walking or jogging, 6 times a week. Continue to increase intensity by picking up your pace, or working at a higher incline, or increase your level on a cardio machine.
Week 5	Perform 2 days of steady-state cardio for 45 minutes each time; perform 2 days of interval cardio.	Perform 3 days of steady-state cardio for 45 minutes each time; perform 2 days of interval cardio.	Perform 4 days of steady-state cardio for 60 minutes each time; perform 2 days of interval cardio.
Week 6	Perform 2 days of steady-state cardio for 45 minutes each time; perform 2 days of interval cardio. Try to increase intensity.	Perform 3 days of steady-state cardio for 45 minutes each time; perform 2 days of interval cardio. Try to increase intensity.	Perform 4 days of steady-state cardio for 60 minutes each time; perform 2 days of interval cardio. Try to increase intensity.

Cardio Workout	Beginner	Intermediate	Advanced
Week 7	Perform 2 days of steady-state cardio for 45 minutes each time; perform 2 days of interval cardio. Try to increase intensity.	Perform 3 days of steady-state cardio for 45 minutes each time; perform 2 days of interval cardio. Try to increase intensity.	Perform 4 days of steady-state cardio for 60 minutes each time; perform 2 days of interval cardio. Try to increase intensity.
Week 8	Perform 2 days of steady-state cardio for 45 minutes each time; perform 2 days of interval cardio. Try to increase intensity.	Perform 3 days of steady-state cardio for 45 minutes each time; perform 2 days of interval cardio. Try to increase intensity.	Perform 4 days of steady-state cardio for 60 minutes each time; perform 2 days of interval cardio. Try to increase intensity.
Week 9	Perform 3 days of steady-state cardio for 45 minutes each time; perform 2 days of interval cardio. Try to increase intensity.	Perform 3 days of steady-state cardio for 45–60 minutes each time; perform 2 days of interval cardio. Try to increase intensity.	Perform 4 days of steady-state cardio for 60 minutes each time; perform 2 days of interval cardio. Try to increase intensity.
Week 10	Perform 3 days of steady-state cardio for 45 minutes each time; perform 2 days of interval cardio. Try to increase intensity.	Perform 4 days of steady-state cardio for 45–60 minutes each time; perform 2 days of interval cardio. Try to increase intensity.	Perform 3 days of steady-state cardio for 60 minutes each time; perform 3 days of interval cardio. Try to increase intensity.
Week 11	Perform 3 days of steady-state cardio for 45–60 minutes each time; perform 2 days of interval cardio. Try to increase intensity.	Perform 3 days of steady-state cardio for 45–60 minutes each time; perform 3 days of interval cardio. Try to increase intensity.	Perform 2 days of steady-state cardio for 60 minutes each time; perform 4 days of interval cardio. Try to increase intensity.
Week 12	Perform 2 days of steady-state cardio for 60 minutes each time; perform 3 days of interval cardio. Try to increase intensity.	Perform 2 days of steady-state cardio for 45–60 minutes each time; perform 4 days of interval cardio. Try to increase intensity.	Perform 1 day of steady-state cardio for 60 minutes; perform 5 days of interval cardio. Try to increase intensity.

you burn more calories and fat, improve your cardiovascular fitness, increase your speed, and expand your workout options.

Here is how we recommend that you do your interval cardio (this works best if you have access to a cardio machine with a speedometer):

Warm up:	3 minutes at 3–4 mph, or at a pace where you can talk easily
Speed up:	5 minutes at 5–6 mph, or at a pace where it takes little effort to talk
Slow down:	1 minute at 3–4 mph
Speed up:	3 minutes at 6–7 mph, or at a pace where it takes more effort to talk
Slow down:	1 minute at 3–4 mph
Speed up:	3 minutes at 7–8 mph, or at a pace where it takes some more effort to talk
Slow down:	1 minute at 3–4 mph
Speed up:	3 minutes at 8–9 mph, or at a pace where talking is starting to get challenging
Slow down:	1 minute at 3–4 mph
Speed up:	3 minutes at 8–9 mph
Slow down:	1 minute at 3–4 mph
Speed up:	1 minute, as fast as you can
Cool down:	2 minutes at 3–4 mph

Cardio Training Guidelines

● Wear a heart rate monitor. This device allows you to gauge your heart rate continuously. Many modern heart rate monitors will actually sound an alarm if you fall below your target heart-rate zone. Try to keep your heart rate between 80 percent and 85 percent of its maximum, so that your body will tap into its fat stores for energy and work at an efficient capacity. To determine your maximum heart rate, subtract your age from 220. Calculating 80 percent and 85 percent of this number provides you with your target heart-rate zone.

● Select any form of cardio exercise: walking, jogging, running, cycling, or swimming or use a cardiovascular machine at the gym, including the treadmill, stair climber, stationary bicycle, or elliptical machine. Choose an activity that you like, so that you won't have an excuse not to do it. The harder and longer you work out at your chosen activity, the more calories you'll burn, regardless of the type of workout.

● If you have access to a cardio machine, such as a treadmill or stationary bike, you can control your intervals by pushing a button to change the level of resistance or speed up your pace. The

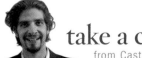

take a cue
from Cast Member Aaron Semmel

Learn how to love to sweat. I always tell people, "Picture that sweat as your fat melting off your body." You'll learn to love exercise (and love sweating) if you hold that image in your mind.

controls on the machine can time your intervals for you.

- Regardless of your fitness level, devote the first 4 weeks of exercise to steady-state cardio only, in order to condition your heart and lungs for higher intensity interval training later in the program.

- Focus on the quality of your workout and encourage yourself to push harder each time.

- Vary your workouts with different forms of cardio to maintain your interest and enthusiasm—even invite a friend to train with you.

- Use the 12-week program as a guide only. If you feel like you can do more or even less than what is prescribed for a particular week, adjust your exercise accordingly. Listen to your body.

- Always consult with your physician prior to beginning any exercise program. Don't start without his or her approval!

- One more piece of advice: Take this program a day at a time, or else you'll get overwhelmed by its totality. It's the effort you put forth on a day-to-day basis that brings you closer to your goal. Every step you take is progress toward uncovering sexy curves and toned muscles!

- Consider yoga, no matter how much you weigh. Yoga helps you get in touch with, and appreciate, your body and what it can do.

- For more efficient fat-burning, consider doing your cardio first thing in the morning—before breakfast. Your body is low on stored carbohydrates then and will tap into fat for energy more readily. A similar option is to perform your cardio workout after your circuit workout. Circuit training burns up stored carbohydrate first; afterward, when you switch to cardio, your body calls on stored fat since your carbohydrate reserve is depleted.

- Try pool training as a great way to burn calories. It's also easy on your joints. The trick is to keep moving in the water—swim laps, walk in the water, or tread water in the deep end. Use some pool toys, too, such as a floating device that allows you to kick your way across the pool or a pool buoy that you can place between your legs, letting them rest while you work on your upper body.

The Fat-Burning Circuit Workout

The second component of the plan is a *circuit training program.* For those of you who aren't familiar with the term, this means that you perform one set of each exercise for 1 minute, then immediately move to the next exercise with only 5 to 8 seconds of rest in between, alternating the muscle groups you work. In other words, you start by working your chest, then move on to your legs, then on to your shoulders, and so forth. This ap-

take a cue
from Cast Member Pete Thomas

I learned that burning 3,500 calories burns away a pound of fat, so while I was on the ranch, my goal was to burn that amount of calories each day so that I'd lose a pound a day.

Exercise Routine for the Fat-Burning Circuit Workout

In the following routine, beginners should use lighter weights; intermediate and advanced exercisers can handle heavier weights, hence the lower number of repetitions.

Exercises	Beginner—Repetitions	Intermediate—Repetitions	Advanced—Repetitions
Push-Ups	12-15	10-12	6-10
Body Weight Squat	12-15	10-12	6-10
Shoulder Press	12-15	10-12	6-10
Body Weight Squat—Repeat	12-15	10-12	6-10
Biceps Curl	12-15	10-12	6-10
Walking Lunges	5 minutes	5 minutes	5 minutes
Chair Dips	12-15	10-12	6-10
Dumbbell Row	12-15	10-12	6-10
Standard Lunges	12-15	10-12	6-10
Abdominal Crunches	7 minutes	7 minutes	7 minutes
Stretching—Cool Down			

proach to exercising taxes your energy systems to create body-firming muscle and increase aerobic capacity, all while reducing body fat.

You'll be on the move constantly during these workouts.

The intensity of this workout is kept high because you're barely resting between sets. For that reason, you'll be using lighter weights than you may have used in a conventional strength-training or weight-lifting program.

take a cue
from Cast Member Ryan Kelly

Mix it up. I do kickboxing, yoga, the revolving stair-climbing machine, weight training, and the elliptical trainer. I like to try things I've never done before.

Important

■ As you add more cardio sessions week by week, you may do your cardio after your circuit training. This sequence accentuates fat loss. Following your circuit routine, your body is low on stored carbohydrate (glycogen). Consequently, your body will tap into its fat stores to help burn energy.

■ Beginners should perform the circuit only once per session. After 2 weeks, begin performing the circuit twice. Intermediate exercisers should perform the circuit twice; after 2 weeks, perform the circuit three times. Advanced exercisers should perform the circuit three times. Most exercises have an advanced variation. Beginners and intermediate exercisers should progress to using the advanced variation when they feel stronger.

■ Drink plenty of water before, during, and after exercise to prevent dehydration. Keep in mind that hydration increases fat burning.

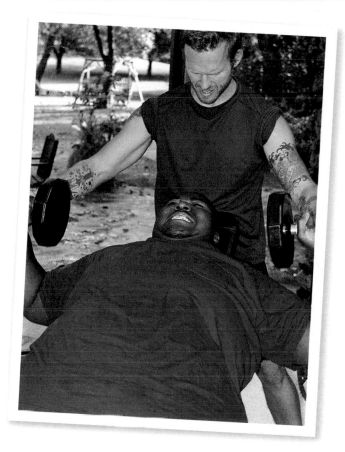

Circuit Training Guidelines

● Wear a heart rate monitor when circuit training and keep your heart rate in its fat-burning zone during your routine.

● Warm up for 5 minutes by walking, marching, or jogging in place.

● Get equipped. The exercises use either your own body weight or dumbbells. Have on hand sets of dumbbells weighing 5, 10, 15, 20, and 25 pounds so that you can gradually increase the weights you use.

● Have on hand a clock or watch with a second hand. The exercises are performed in time intervals; therefore, you'll need to time yourself.

● When performing an exercise, select a weight that allows you to perform only the specified number of reps for your routine. If the exercise feels too easy, progressively increase the weights. Depending on your strength level, you may need to purchase even heavier dumbbells.

● Perform this workout program three times per week, resting at least a day between circuit workouts.

Exercise Instructions

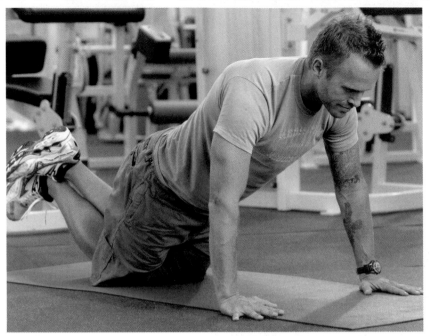

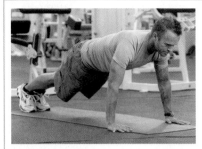

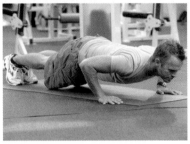

Advanced version

It is more challenging to keep your legs straight and your toes tucked under your feet. To begin, lie face-down with your palms on the floor, placed shoulder-width apart, and your feet extended; make sure your legs are parallel to each other. Straighten your arms as you push your body off the floor. Next, lower your body until your chest touches the floor. Keep your back straight and your knees off the floor. Repeat the exercise for the recommended number of repetitions for your level.

Push-Ups

This well-known exercise is great for shaping your chest and arms, plus building overall body strength. Lie facedown with your palms on the floor, placed shoulder-width apart, and your knees bent with your ankles crossed.

Straighten your arms as you push your body up off the floor. Try not to bend or arch your back as you push up. Next, slowly lower your chest toward the floor. Bend your arms and keep

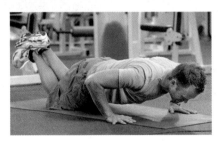

your palms in their fixed position. Repeat the exercise for the recommended number of repetitions for your level.

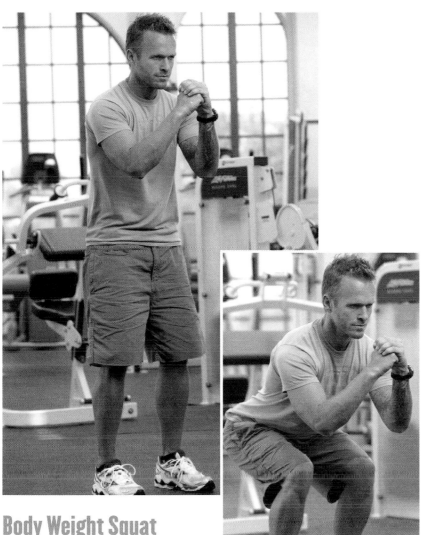

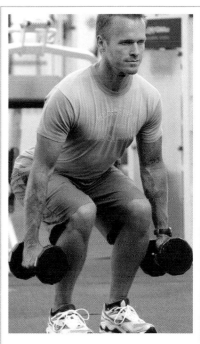

Advanced version

This version is performed in the same manner as the body weight squat, except that you will hold a dumbbell in each hand at your sides. With your back erect and your head up, slowly bend your knees until your thighs are nearly parallel to the floor. Straighten your legs and return to the starting position. Repeat the exercise for the recommended number of reps for your level.

Body Weight Squat

This exercise works the thighs, hips, and buttocks and requires no special equipment. To begin, stand with your feet about shoulder-width apart and your arms in front of you, as shown. Keeping your back straight, squat down until your thighs are about parallel to the floor. Press up from your heels and return to the starting position. Repeat the exercise for the recommended number of reps for your level.

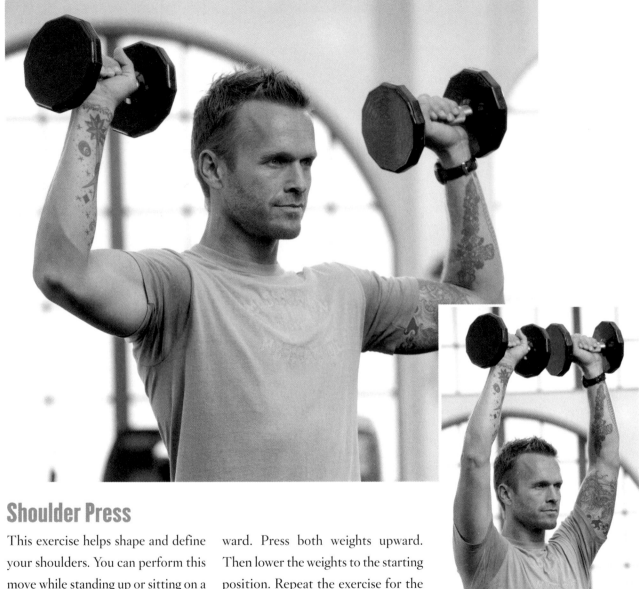

Shoulder Press

This exercise helps shape and define your shoulders. You can perform this move while standing up or sitting on a chair. To begin, grasp two dumbbells with an overhand grip and hold them at shoulder level, palms facing for- ward. Press both weights upward. Then lower the weights to the starting position. Repeat the exercise for the recommended number of reps for your level.

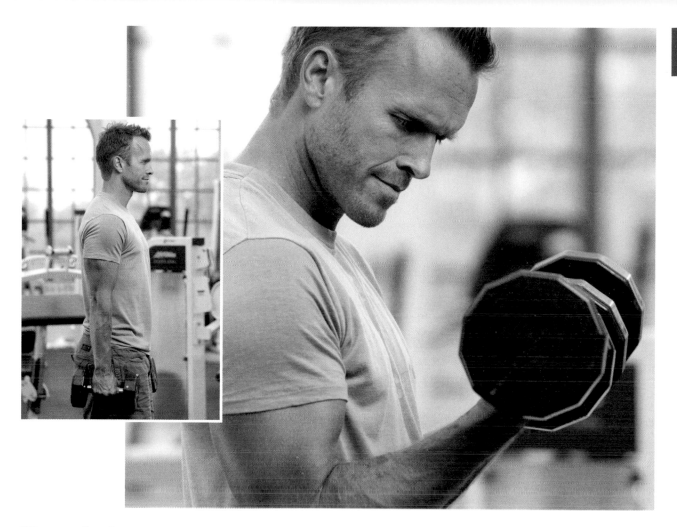

Biceps Curl

This exercise tones the front of your upper arms. To begin, stand with your feet about shoulder-width apart. With your arms at your sides, hold a dumbbell in each hand, palms facing front or inward. Flex at the elbows and curl the weights up toward your shoulders and tense your biceps at the top of the exercise. Slowly lower the dumbbells back to the starting position. Repeat the exercise for the recommended number of reps for your level.

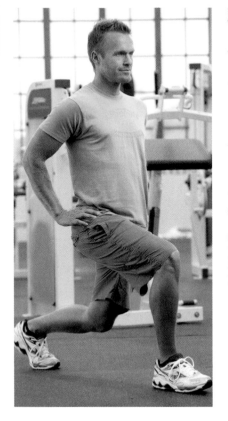
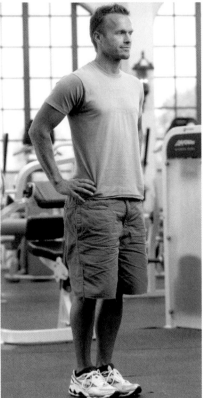
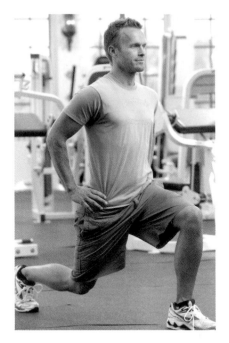

Walking Lunges

This exercise is an excellent move for shaping your legs and buttocks. For walking lunges, you'll need more space in which you can move around.

While keeping your back straight, step forward on your right leg as far as possible, until your right thigh is about parallel to the floor. Then bring your left leg forward to meet your right leg.

Next, step forward on your left leg as far as possible, until your left thigh is about parallel to the floor. Then bring your right leg forward to meet your left leg. Continue the exercise in this manner by walking forward for a full 5 minutes.

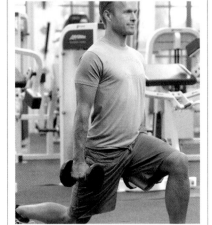

Advanced version

Hold a dumbbell in each hand at your sides. Perform the exercise as previously directed.

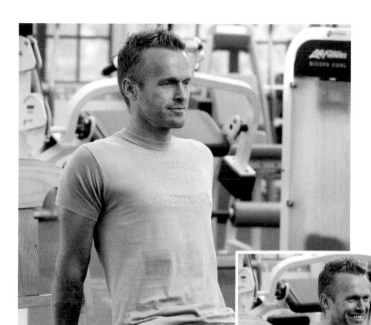

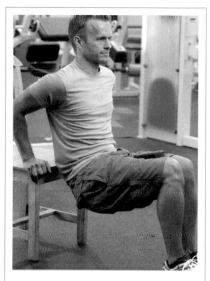

Advanced version

To make this exercise more challenging, place a dumbbell or other weight on your lap. Perform the exercise as previously directed.

Chair Dips

Chair dips are an easy, do-anywhere exercise for firming up the backs of your upper arms, where age and neglect can result in a flabby appearance. All you need is a sturdy chair for this exercise.

To begin, sit on the edge of the chair. Grasp the edge of the chair's seat, making sure your forearms and fingers are pointing forward. Your legs should be extended out in front of you, ankles crossed, with your heels supporting your lower body. Slowly bend your elbows to lower your hips to the floor. Push yourself back up by straightening your arms. Repeat the exercise for the recommended number of repetitions for your level.

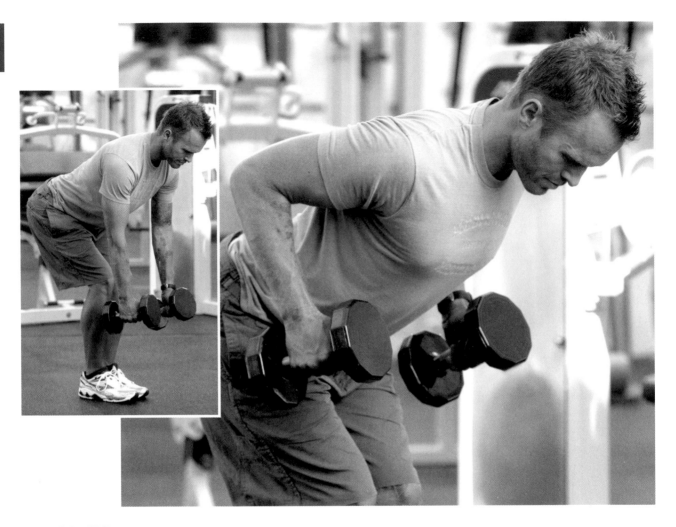

Dumbbell Row

This exercise is designed to tone and sculpt your upper and midback. Grasp a pair of dumbbells using an overhand grip. Bend your knees slightly. With your back in its natural alignment, bend 90 degrees at the waist. Pull the dumbbells into the sides of your midsection. Contract your back muscles. Slowly lower the weights to the starting position. Repeat the exercise for the recommended number of repetitions for your level.

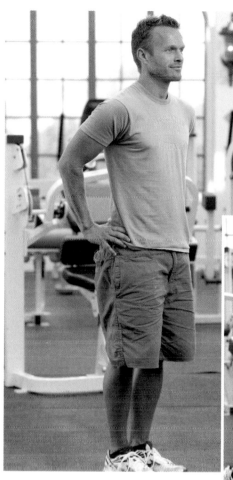

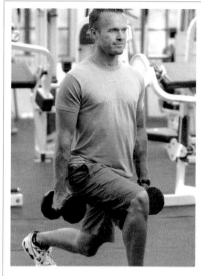

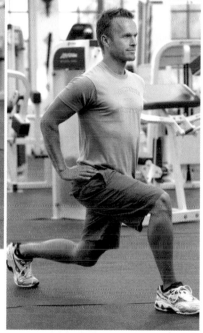

Advanced version

Take a dumbbell in each hand and hold them along each side of your body. Perform the exercise as previously explained.

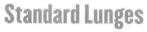

Standard Lunges

This exercise is great for firming up your thighs and buttocks. Begin with both legs together. Step forward about 2 feet with one leg until your front thigh is nearly parallel to the floor. Concentrate on getting a good stretch and on keeping your back straight.

Next, push yourself back to the starting position and continue lunging forward on the same leg for the required number of repetitions. Switch legs and repeat the exercise.

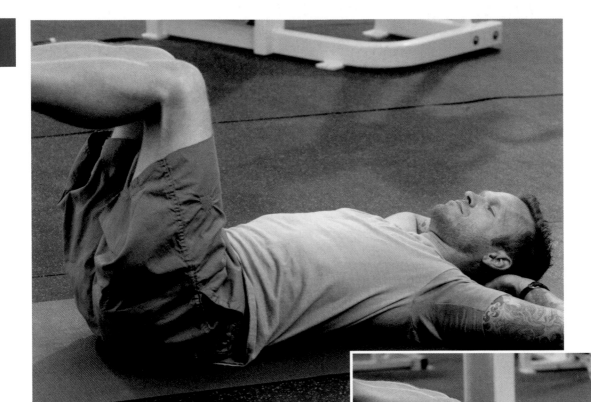

Abdominal Crunches

This exercise will help transform a soft tummy into flat, toned abs. Lie on your back on a soft surface such as a carpet or exercise mat, and place your hands behind your head. You may place your legs in a table-top position with your thighs perpendicular to the floor and your knees bent, or simply run your legs up a wall. Using the strength of your abdominal muscles, lift your upper body from the floor toward your legs. Tense your abdominal muscles at the top of the exercise. Lower and repeat. Exercise your abs in this manner for a total of 7 minutes.

Stretch Series

End every circuit and cardio workout with the following static stretches for all major muscles, holding each stretch for 15 to 30 seconds without bouncing.

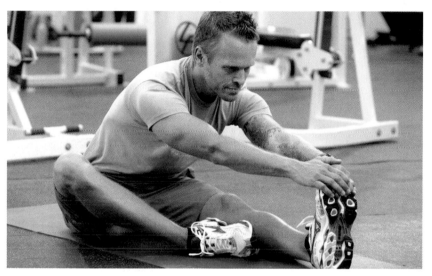

Hamstring Stretch

Sit on the floor with your legs slightly apart. Bend forward from your waist, keeping your knees straight. Try to reach your fingers toward your toes. Hold for 15 to 30 seconds. As you get more flexible, try to grab the tops of your shoes.

Quadriceps Stretch

Hold on to a wall or sturdy table for support with your left hand. Bring your right foot toward your back and hold it with your right hand. Keep your knees slightly bent. Gently pull up and back on your foot, stretching your thigh. Hold for 15 to 30 seconds. Repeat the stretch with your other leg.

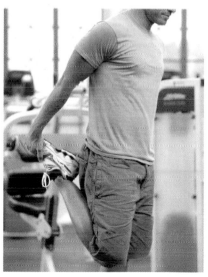

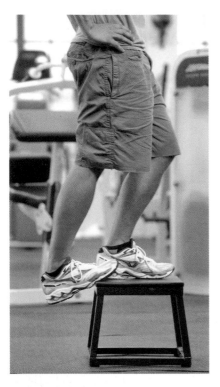

Calf Stretch

Stand on a stair. Move one foot back toward the edge of the stair, so that only your toes are touching the edge. Lower your heel toward the ground until you feel a good stretch in your calf. Hold for 15 to 30 seconds. Repeat the stretch with your other leg.

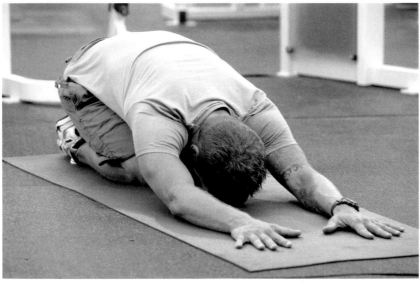

Child's Pose

Kneel down on the floor and sit back toward your heels, while extending your arms forward. Rest your forehead on the floor. Stretch your back and relax your neck and shoulders. Hold for 15 to 30 seconds.

Mix It and Match It

If you're among the millions of people who watched *The Biggest Loser* each week, you saw the cast members participate in a varied exercise menu, in addition to cardio and strength training. They hiked, they did yoga, they swam, and they played sports. The lesson in what you watched is that it's not a good idea to get stuck in a rut with a single activity week after week. A mix of different types of exercise stimulates your body and mind, helps you avoid injuries, and perhaps best of all, keeps you motivated.

Quite probably, some of the activities you like best—tennis, racquetball, volleyball, basketball, or dancing—actually complement conventional cardio because they involve intense bursts of muscle activity. Those bursts force your muscles to react quickly, and that improves your agility and coordination. What's more, your muscles get a good workout in the process.

Mixing and matching a variety of activities is often called cross-training, and it's an excellent way to achieve all-around fitness. One specific benefit of cross-training is the cardio benefit that carries over to other activities and sports. The fitness you gain by walking or running, for example, will let you bike, swim, and hike farther or play tennis, racquetball, or basketball longer. Or if you strength-train, the muscle strength you achieve will give you power for other sports.

Cross-training brings more muscles into motion, and that contributes to building a stronger, healthier body. Find several different types of activities you enjoy, even some

10 Great Reasons to Stay Active

If you're like most people, you start exercising with one or two goals in mind: losing weight, or shaping up. But there are many more benefits. Once you become more active and keep at it, you'll find yourself better for it in more ways than one.

1. People who exercise live longer, on average, than people who don't.
2. Active people have a lower risk of dying from heart disease and stroke, and they're less likely to get high blood pressure.
3. The more active you are, the lower your risk of colon cancer.
4. The less active you are, the higher your risk of getting type 2 diabetes. If you already have type 2 diabetes, exercise can lower your blood sugar levels.
5. For people with arthritis, moderate exercise helps reduce joint swelling and pain and improves mobility.
6. Strength-building exercise helps counter bone loss (osteoporosis).
7. Exercise makes you "functionally fit," meaning that it's easier for you to carry groceries, do chores, and independently perform many other activities of daily life.
8. Because of the calming effect of exercise, active people are less depressed, and depressed people often feel better after they start exercising.
9. Exercise can save you money. If you can prevent serious—and costly—medical conditions such as heart disease, cancer, and osteoporosis, you will have more money for your other needs.
10. Exercise can be fun! Many of the activities you did for play as a child count as exercise. Dancing fast, walking your dog, bicycling, and gardening all strengthen your heart and lungs.

that get you outdoors. Consider joining a running group, cycling group, hiking club, swim team, or rock-climbing classes. Your options are endless. Not only will you get in better shape, you'll start interacting with an entirely new group of people you would not have met before—people who can further motivate you and inspire you in your fitness endeavors and lifestyle change.

When it comes to fitness, variation through cross-training is the key to staying power and continued results. To become your own Biggest Loser, make it a point to live a life full of challenging, stimulating, and fun activities.

You Can Do It!

Right now, as you've finished reading this chapter, you may be thinking that you're being asked to do a lot. You are! But if you can stay with this program on a regular basis, your body will start burning stored fat very rapidly. Please remember that this is a fail-proof program for improving your body, your shape, and your health.

It's human nature to listen to those negative voices inside you that tell you "you can't." You've got to get in the habit of overriding that negativity with positive energy. You have power and potential you don't know you have! It's just a matter of reaching deep down inside you and testing your limits. You don't know how far you can go with exercise or anything else until you go for it. You are stronger than you think!

Well into season one, the remaining cast members were faced with one of their most difficult physical challenges ever. As they filed into the exercise room, they saw what initially frightened them: a row of six spinning bicycles, each with their name on it, set up and ready to go, with a big clock hovering in the room.

Caroline Rhea announced that the cast members had 4 hours to travel as many miles as they could on the bikes. Whoever rode the most miles by midnight would win the challenge. The prize was immunity from being eliminated that day, even if the winner had gained weight, plus a shopping spree for a new wardrobe.

There were gasps. Gary started pacing back and forth. Drea, who had taken a lot of spin classes before, thought to herself, "I know what 45 minutes on a spin bike feels like. How on earth do you last 4 hours on that seat?"

Lisa felt panicky. She disliked spinning, preferring

take a cue
from Cast Member Drea Baptiste

Most of the people I've met since being on the show have been so encouraging and so positive. But there are a few who say we were successful only because we had personal trainers. To them, I say, "You have a trainer in your house, too, and you don't have to pay hundreds of dollars for him or her." All of those video or DVD exercise recordings you have in your house contain your personal trainers, such as Billy Blanks, Denise Austin, Jane Fonda, or other well-known exercise personalities. Just like Bob and Jillian, they can stand there and tell you what to do, but it won't work until you do it. So just pop in the videotape or DVD, and get to work!

strength training instead. "Of course, my blood pressure, my anxiety, everything went through the roof when I saw what we had to do. But I wanted to prove to myself that I could complete something."

Can you imagine how grueling it must have been to ride an exercise bike for 4 hours straight, in the evening, right up until the clock struck midnight?

They all took their places, then took off. The first few minutes seemed effortless; it didn't feel so bad. Before long though, butts started getting sore. Legs were feeling mushy. Quads were burning. Sweat was dripping. This was hard work, and every minute seemed like an eternity. Everyone was feeling the exact same pain, but they were pushing through it, testing their own limits, all going for the prize.

Pedaling feverishly, Gary began to pull away from the pack and the rest fell behind, losing their legs but not the will to continue. No one could catch up with Gary, though. Collectively, the cast members agreed to take periodic breaks. But Gary did not get off the bike even once. He got so far ahead that Drea, Kelly (Minner), and Ryan decided that they would just use the challenge to work off pounds for the next day's weigh in.

Gary wasn't going to give up—or give in. He was untouchable and unbeatable. To no one's surprise, he ended

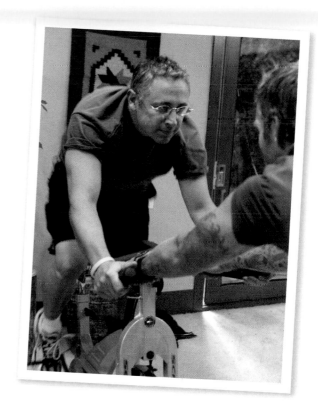

up the winner, logging in an impressive 79 miles.

Despite the odds, Lisa spun her heart out that night—and came in second after Gary—pedaling 69.7 miles.

By the end of the challenge, they dragged their exhausted selves from their bikes, and even though Gary won, the other cast members felt pretty good about what they had accomplished. Imagine this: It was Mo Walker's

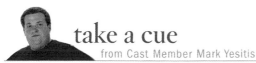

take a cue
from Cast Member Mark Yesitis

For me it's calories in, calories out. That's why I like cardio machines. The digital readouts tell me exactly how many calories I'm burning with each exercise session. If I want to burn 1,500 calories—which is nearly half a pound of fat—the machine counts those calories for me. As long as I'm burning more calories during the day than I eat, I'm going to lose weight.

first time on a spinning bike. He normally worked out on a recumbent bike only. When it was all said and done, Mo pedaled a respectable 40 miles and burned 5,000 calories that night. Not bad for someone who had never been on a spin bike before! As Mo said afterward, "I was really proud of myself for what I accomplished tonight. Although it might be a couple of days before I look at a spin bike again, I definitely plan on making this part of my training regimen."

Early on in the season, Gary would often complain, "I don't have it; I'm not going to do it." He was initially the "I can't guy," someone who had been known to get weak, give up, even stop in the middle of spin classes. Ultimately, he had to break through that mental barrier. This challenge smashed it. At the end of the challenge, Gary had this to say: "I was very surprised about my own ability. I wanted to prove to myself that I was strong." "I can't" was no longer in Gary's vocabulary.

Of course, everyone was a winner that night. The moral of this challenge is that you too can summon up power and strength you didn't know you had, enjoy the ride along the way, and keep your eye on your own prize—a trim, healthy, fit body. In the end, a combination of determination and a can-do attitude will get you to the finish line.

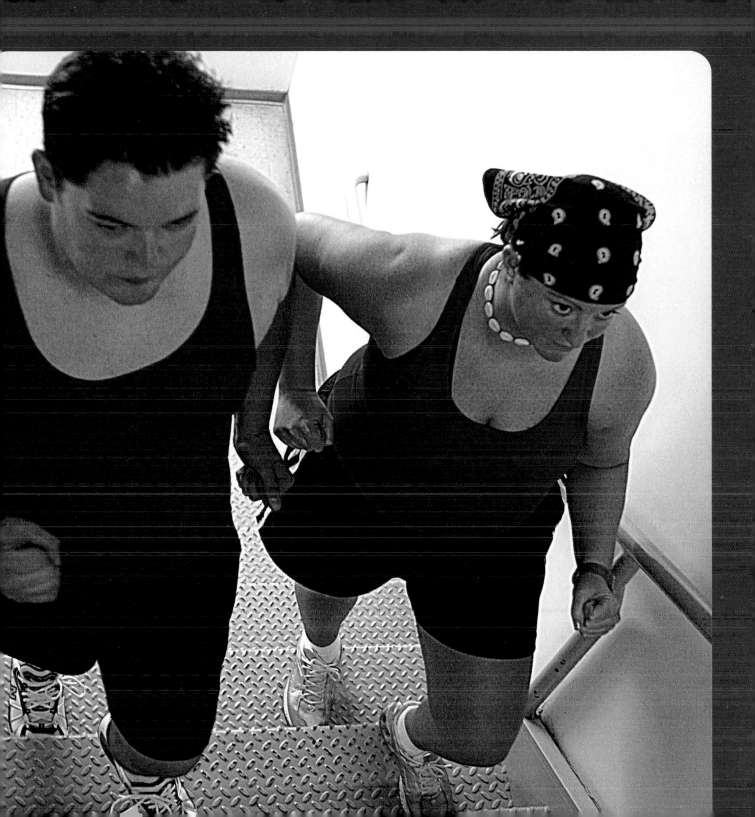

5 Winning Strategies
FROM THE
BIGGEST LOSERS

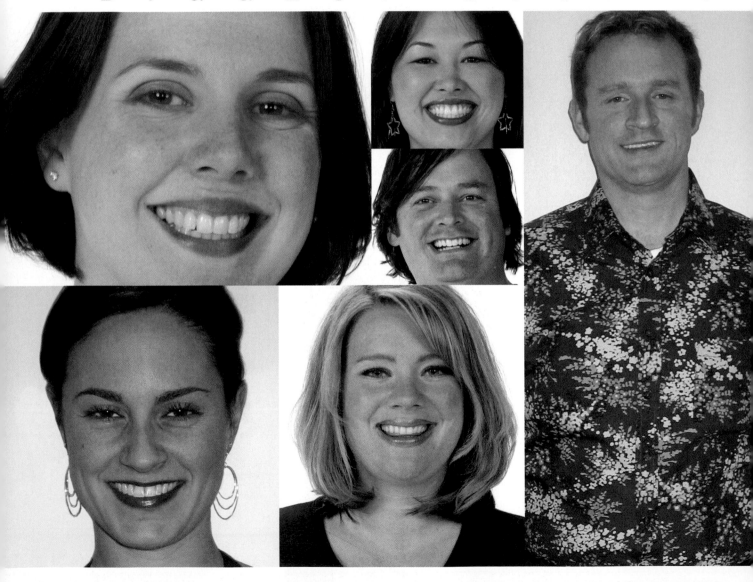

In their formerly fat lives, the cast members of *The Biggest Loser* gained weight because they each had a lot of small bad habits. Ryan Benson used to eat gobs of food in his car. Kathryn Murphy was prone to bingeing at night. Matt Hoover was a heavy beer drinker. Jeff Levine would nosh to keep himself awake during 36-hour residency rotations. Lisa Andreone helped herself to a lot of second and third helpings. Gary Deckman rarely exercised. Mark Yesitis would knock back gallon after gallon of cola. Mo Walker loved to feast on his mom's home-cooked fried chicken. Those little habits added up to big pounds.

But the opposite is also true. Lots of little *good* habits can help you lose lots of weight. You can shed pounds by making some simple adjustments in the way you eat, exercise, think, and act. Make these small adjustments enough, and they'll slowly but surely transform your behavior. Before you know it, they'll take hold, and you will have developed some strong healthy habits that will help you become slim and fit.

Like you, the cast members have had their ups and downs, their struggles, and their temptations. But the strategies they learned on the ranch are so simple and realistic that the cast members easily incorporated them into their daily and weekly routines—and they can see keeping up on these good habits for the rest of their lives. Check out their strategies below for help and inspiration, and see what in-the-trenches Biggest Losers and trainers advise for forever-lean, healthy living. Taken together, their tips might just add up to some impressive weight loss for you, too.

Mind-Set & Motivation

Use your brain to outsmart all those bad habits that undermine your ability to lose weight. Changing your body starts with changing your mind. Get rid of self-defeating "I can't" thoughts. Stop turning to food to relieve stress, and make *yourself* a priority. In other words, start thinking like a Biggest Loser if you want to succeed. Here's how.

Jillian Michaels

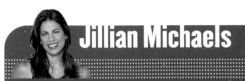

■ If you're prone to emotional overeating, identify what is happening psychologically, deal with that situation, verbalize your feelings, and address that issue rather than turn to food.

Mo Walker

At the ranch, I learned a lot about diet and exercise, but I would have to say the most important thing I learned was to believe in myself. I know I can do it, no matter how insurmountable things may seem. I can dig down deep inside and I can do it.

Aaron Semmel

Never, ever give up on the thought of a "thin you." Always have the thin-you vision in your head. It's attainable.

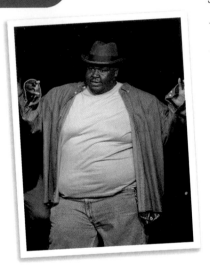

Lisa Andreone

■ I've heard that it takes 12 days to start a new habit. So if you can just **stick it out for 12 days,** then you're on your way.

■ Start gradually. I always tell people to **try the diet part for 2 weeks,** without the exercise. Then after the 2 weeks, add a little exercise, twice a week, and continue to **gradually increase the number of workouts** you do each week.

Matt Kamont

Think of each piece of junk food that you re-move from your house as equating to a pound of fat you lose. If you toss out 50 junk food items, that's 50 pounds.

Seth Word

Expect your mind to be very negative in the beginning. It tells you that you're tired, or that your muscles are burning. Yet that's the time when it is the most important to keep going. When I get those negative thoughts, **I use them as fuel to push through** and force my body to keep going. In other words, when my mind says "stop," that's a signal to go.

Shannon Mullen

Think of everything that is positive in your life, especially your family and your children. I had my daughter very young. I'm going to be around for a long time. She's almost 12, and I just turned 30. We're basically growing up to-gether. I need to make sure that I'm around as long as I can be here for her. Children are such a great motivation.

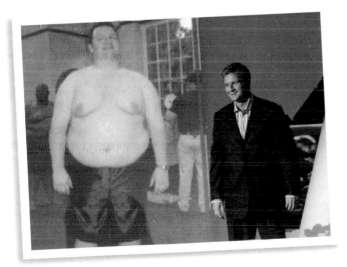

Ryan Benson

Don't get overwhelmed by the amount of weight you need to lose. Take it one day at a time, one pound at a time.

Gary Deckman

Set an example for your family. This whole process for me has been about a lifestyle change. It's not just about going to exercise at the gym and working out. It's not just about the diet. It's about my family. It's about incorporating all of that, the exercise and the diet into my life, **making it fun, making it healthy,** and building for my kids' future in terms of health. If my kids see me doing healthy things, they're going to learn healthy things to do as well and they're going to **continue living in a healthy manner.**

Lizzeth Davalos

Helping others helps me stay motivated. My mother and sister are a big part of my life, and I love to help them with their weight loss.

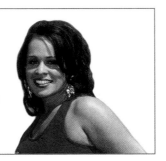

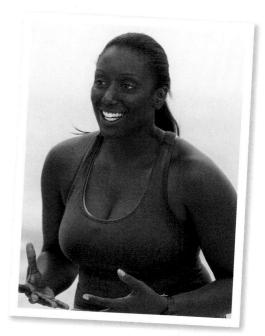

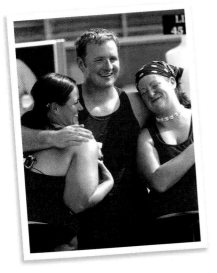

Drea Baptiste

If you can look at yourself in the mirror and say "I'm ready," then seize that moment because you're absolutely ready and there's nothing stopping you. Don't put it off.

Kelly Minner

I've learned to tell people "no." When friends want me to go to happy hour, for instance, I tell them that I'm going to the gym because that's my schedule, and I'm not changing it. It has nothing to do with not wanting to have fun with my friends; it's what I need to do for me, and everything else comes after it.

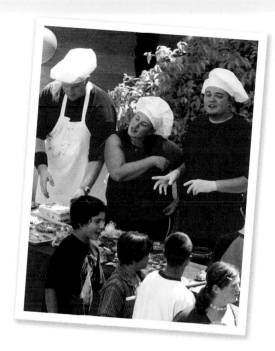

Bob Harper

It is never too late to take charge of your life.

Pete Thomas

Lose weight with a buddy.
Two is always better than one.

Matt Hoover

Each day is a new day. It doesn't matter how hard you worked yesterday or how hard you didn't work yesterday, you have to pick it back up and keep going.

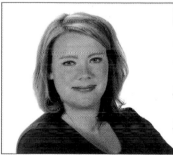

Ryan Kelly

Life is too short to spend it overweight and miserable.

Food Choices

Obviously, if you want to lose weight and get in shape, you need to save calories where you can, while making the healthiest food choices possible in the proper portions. Here's an inside look at what has worked best for the cast members of *The Biggest Loser.*

Bob Harper

- If it grows out of the ground or you can pick it off a tree, chances are that it's good for you.
- Add a little Crystal Light to your water for a sweeter taste.

Lisa Andreone

If I eat chocolate chip cookies, my butt is in the gym the next day working out.

Kathryn Murphy

If you love chocolate, buy diet chocolate Fudgsicles. They're only 40 calories a piece and taste great.

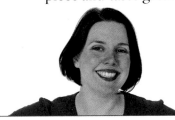

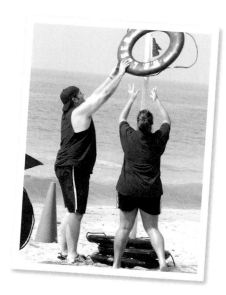

Mark Yesitis

My biggest downfall was cola. On a hot summer day, I could drink 2 liters easily. That's loads of calories. I've learned to substitute Diet Rite cola. It has zero sodium, zero calories, and zero carbs. That's all my daughters are drinking now. There will be no regular colas in my house anymore.

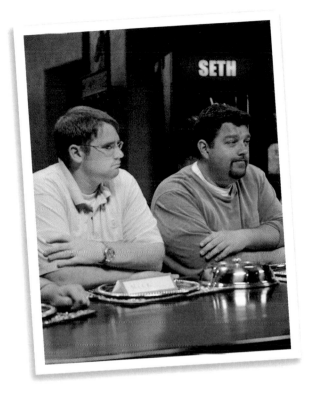

Jillian Michaels

- Losing weight is not about starving yourself; it's about eating what you want, with certain modifications.
- It's okay if you don't like spinach or broccoli. You don't have to eat it. Find what you like and make it work for you.

Dana DeSilvio

Try to avoid sugar. It gives you cravings for more food.

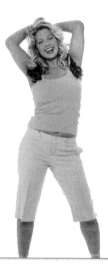

Seth Word

Have protein with your carbohydrates at meals. That way, your meal breaks down more slowly in your body, and you won't burn out so fast and lose energy.

Kelly Minner

- Vary your caloric intake to keep your body guessing. One week you may eat 1,200 calories a day; another week, 1,500 calories.
- Do not deprive or restrict yourself too much or you won't succeed. Allow yourself to have some things you want. It's all about portion control.
- Rather than buy food at a bake sale to raise funds, make a financial donation instead.

Food Choices (continued)

Mo Walker

In the grocery store, stay away from the middle of the store. That's where all the processed food is. Shop in the outer aisles where the fresh fruits and vegetables are.

Matt Hoover

■ If you're throwing down a bunch of beer on Friday or Saturday night, that's enough to negate the whole week's work.

■ I can eat more healthy food than I can eat junk food. I can have an entire day's worth of food for 1,500 calories.

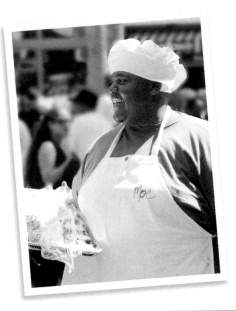

Dave Fioravanti

Establish an eating routine in which you eat every 3 hours. You'll keep your hunger in check.

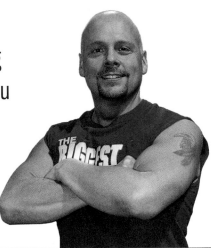

Jeff Levine

■ I have always loved lox and bagels. But because bagels are so high in calories, I now substitute Wasa bread. I can eat five slices of Wasa bread and it adds up to only 100 calories, with very little fat or carbohydrate. I put fat-free cream cheese on the Wasa bread with the onions and lox, and I don't even taste the difference.

■ Cheese can be one of the hardest foods to give up to lose weight. If you love cheese, substitute its low-fat or nonfat counterpart. That way, you can feel good about eating cheese again.

Shannon Mullen

If you're a bread lover, learn to love Ezekiel bread. It is very dense, chewy, and filling and is made with sprouted wheat, spelt, barley, and lentils. **It's a healthy carbohydrate choice.** I can get people in my family to eat it without a problem.

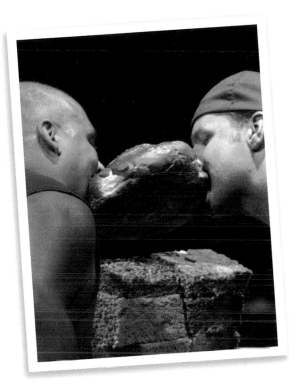

Pete Thomas

Stay hydrated with lots of water to keep your body burning fat. If you hit a plateau, it may be because you're dehydrated.

Jen Kersey

■ Do your grocery shopping in a whole foods store. You'll discover a world of healthy foods you can eat.

■ If you have a sweet tooth, eat fresh pineapple. Its sweetness is unbelievable.

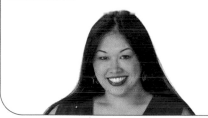

Matt Kamont

■ Don't live in a house without vegetable spray, string cheese, and sugar-free Jell-O.

■ Use the cap from a salad dressing bottle to measure your salad dressing. It equals 1 tablespoon.

Dining Out Strategies

Restaurants don't have to be a dieter's downfall; they can be a dieter's dream—if you're assertive with the waitstaff and know how to order. Here are some tricks the cast members use to avoid some of the common pitfalls of eating out.

Mark Yesitis

■ If your calories for the day don't allow you to eat an entire piece of cheesecake or something else for dessert at a restaurant, eat half of it. Then pour salt on the rest to avoid temptation.

■ Be a pain in the ass in a restaurant. Ask them to use Pam, no butter. It's okay. You're paying them. You're the customer. Change it up. Do what you need to do.

Ryan Kelly

Know the calorie counts of fast foods. For example, I know that a taco at a Mexican fast food restaurant has only 185 calories. So I order a taco.

Matt Kamont

When eating out, always have a salad first. It will dull your appetite.

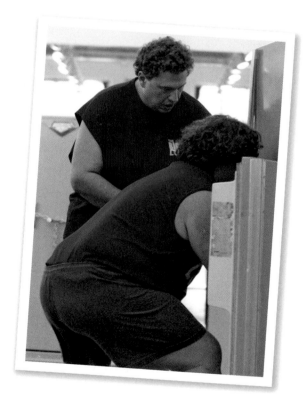

Bob Harper

A great appetizer to order at an Asian restaurant or a sushi bar is edamame, steamed soybeans. They're delicious, and you can fix them at home, too. Just pop them in the microwave for a few seconds, then sprinkle a little sea salt on them, and enjoy.

Aaron Semmel

If you want to lose weight, move away from Chicago. Everything here has mozzarella cheese on it. I'm surprised it doesn't come on ice cream.

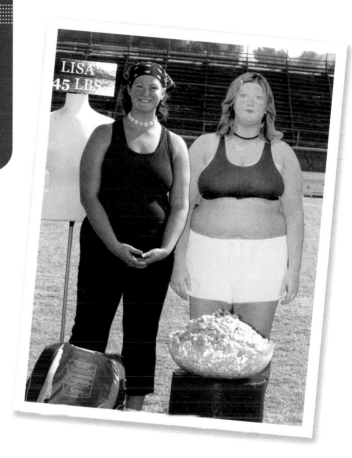

Lisa Andreone

■ Tell the server: Don't even bring out the bread. That's the first request out of my mouth at a restaurant.

■ Sometimes, I will order whatever I want—say lasagna and salad with dressing on the side. However, I will have them bring a to-go box right away. I cut the lasagna in half and put half of the lasagna and half the salad in the box. That way, you still get your lasagna, just not so much of it.

Self-Monitoring

Self-monitoring means observing and recording some aspect of your behavior, such as calorie intake, servings of fruits and vegetables, or exercise sessions, or watching for changes in weight and responding to them quickly. The scientific proof is overwhelming, too: People who "self-monitor" their weight are more successful at losing weight and keeping it off than people who do not self-monitor. They don't just let things go. They take action if their weight gets into an unacceptable range. Here's a look at how some of the Biggest Losers self-monitor their progress.

Bob Harper

Use your food journal to keep track of what triggers you to overeat—negative emotions, stress, a celebration, or being with certain people. Identifying these trigger situations will help you put a stop to them.

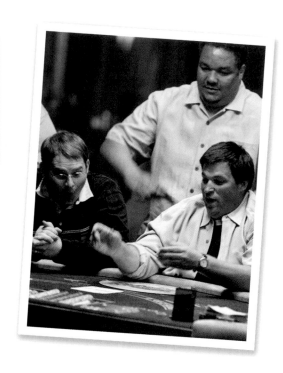

Mark Yesitis

Carry your calorie book with you.
It will fit in your purse or pocket.

Lisa Andreone

In my house, I keep a big cardboard cutout of myself when I weighed 242 pounds. The cutout is a "souvenir" of my participation in season one of *The Biggest Loser.* It reminds me that I never want to look like that again. It's disgusting. I look at that person and ask myself, "How could I ever let myself get like that?"

Ryan Benson

My Biggest Loser ring is fun to have and it means a lot to me. I use it as a reminder of the things I need to be doing, whether it's to drink more water or to turn down an extra piece of bread. Pick a token like a ring or a bracelet, and wear it to remind you to stay on track.

Gary Deckman

I never used to allow a scale in my house. I knew if I was overweight when my clothes got tight or I couldn't cinch my belt. But now I have a scale. It tells me that if I gain a pound or two, it's time to get back on track.

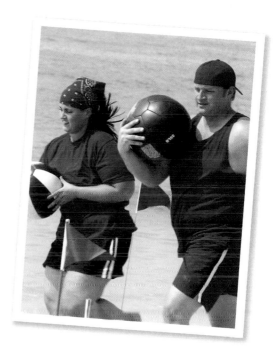

Dave Fioravanti

Buy a few items of clothing that are too expensive to "grow out of." I have a couple of $3,000 sports jackets, for example. If I put them on and feel strangled in them, I'm going to be mad because I won't want to replace them. I just get back on track. It's a lot cheaper.

Exercise Strategies

Nothing helps you lose unsightly body fat faster than exercise. It revs up your metabolism for a better calorie burn, plus reshapes your body to reveal attractive curves and muscles. It keeps you looking and feeling youthful. Even so, about half of all new exercisers quit working out within the first 6 months. How can you stay with it and not become an exercise dropout? Take to heart these tips from the cast members.

 Jillian Michaels

Exercise becomes fun when you become physically capable. When you can look at yourself and say, "I'm a kick-boxer" or "I'm sprinting 11 miles an hour," that's when exercise is fun.

Gary Deckman

Incorporate your family into working out and make it fun. For example, I'm teaching my kids how to play volleyball, and we're doing it on the beach.

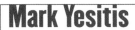

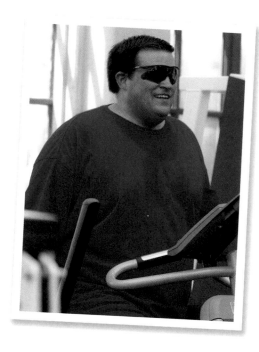

Mark Yesitis

I used to watch 2 hours of TV a day. Now I take that 2 hours and replace it with 2 or 3 hours of exercise.

Lizzeth Davalos

Plan and schedule your exercise sessions a week ahead of time. That way, if something comes up, you can get your workout in.

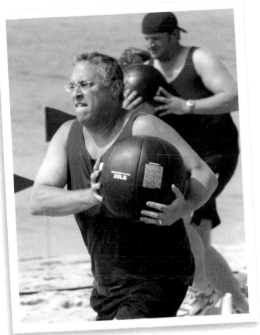

Shannon Mullen

■ Just get it done. When you say you're going to do it later, it doesn't happen and you feel guilty about it.

■ I work at a desk job where I sit all day. There's no need to even leave the building. So I asked myself, "What can I do to become more active while on the job? Is it realistic for me to use the stairs in the morning (I'm on the 11th floor)?" Sure it is!

Mo Walker

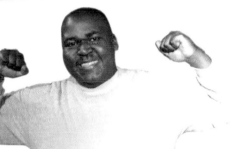

I love to wake up the next morning after a workout feeling sore because I know I am getting healthier.

Seth Word

A big reason why people don't exercise is because they're afraid of what people in the gym will think of them. Don't be afraid to go to the gym because you're already overweight. Push past that. Get off the couch and stop being lazy. Make a commitment to yourself.

Matt Hoover

I think about my relationship with my girlfriend. What better thing can you do for your relationship than go for a walk and talk to each other for a whole hour straight? Set that time aside for both of you—go for a walk and talk and walk at a moderate pace to get the exercise benefits. I'm amazed that it took me this long to figure it out.

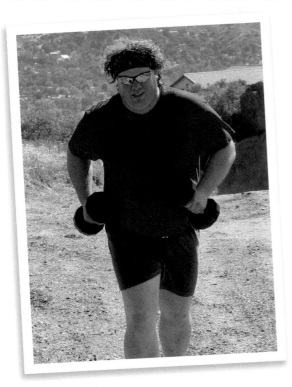

Ryan Kelly

You can have the best trainers in the world, but you're the one who gets out there and does it, not your trainer.

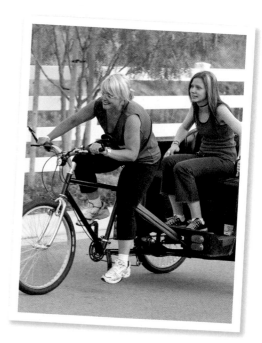

Pete Thomas

Have some healthy carbs like fruit prior to exercising. You'll have more energy to push hard through your workout.

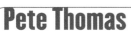

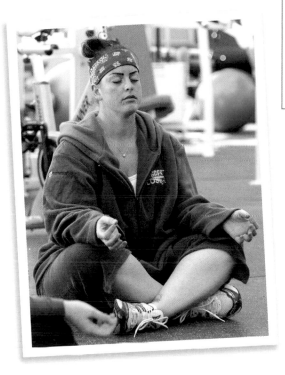

Kelly Minner

■ Find a workout partner. It helps keep you going if there is someone counting on you to be at the gym at a certain time.

■ Switch up your exercise routine from time to time, training your entire body so you don't get into a slump.

Lisa Andreone

Make exercising part of your routine like brushing your teeth. You'll train your body to want to exercise.

Consider adopting these can't-miss tips for losing weight as your own box of tricks. If they worked for the Biggest Losers, they will also work for you. By committing yourself to new lifetime habits and lifestyle changes like these, you'll be able to stay on the wagon and ride all the way to your goal weight.

6 Start Your Own

BIGGEST LOSER
CHALLENGE

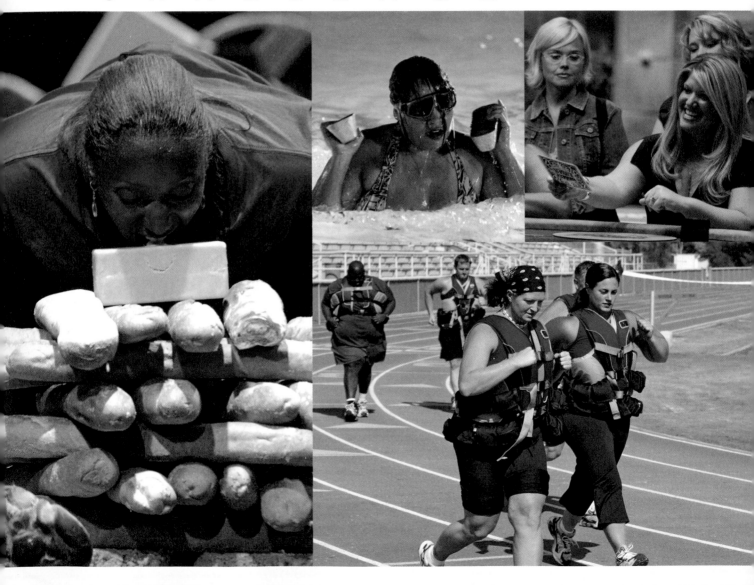

Over the course of two gripping seasons, *The Biggest Loser* gave America an inside, up-close-and-personal look at what it takes to struggle with temptation, resolve long-standing food issues, and yet through it all, lose

pound after pound by eating healthfully and exercising. Each cast member, with their dedication and determination to get healthier, trimmer bodies, inspired an overweight America to get fit. For many cast members, those Americans were right in their own backyards.

Case in point: Dr. Jeff Levine had been treating a patient back home who weighed in at a deadly 430 pounds. "I had to hospitalize this guy several times, all because of medical problems associated with his weight," Jeff explained. "He was always in denial about his weight and would never let me bring it up. If I mentioned his weight, he got mad."

While at the ranch battling to shed his own health-damaging 370 pounds, Jeff received a letter from this particular patient. Jeff could hardly believe the words he was reading: This man wrote that he was so inspired by Jeff's decision to address his own weight that he (the patient) lost 60 pounds!

"That has been a tremendous motivator for me," Jeff said, "to know not only that I am going to help myself and my family, but also that my experience will make me a more effective family physician."

There are more stories like this. Matt Kamont knew from day one that people all over the country would be looking up to him. "I couldn't let them down. If I quit, if I packed my bags, if I decided to not get on that treadmill,

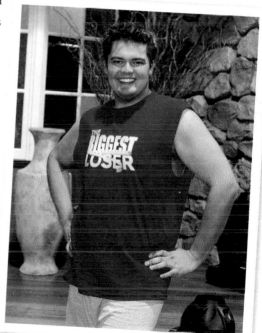

Matt Kamont, after *The Biggest Loser*

I wasn't just hurting myself, I was hurting everyone in America. I did not want to let anyone down."

Matt stayed true to his mission. Once off the ranch, Matt met many, many people who were inspired by his 75-pound weight loss. But perhaps the most inspired were people in his own family. Matt's mother lost more than 20 pounds (and quit smoking after 20 years!). His sister dropped more than 30 pounds. His uncle is now 40 pounds lighter. A former roommate of Matt's shed 25 pounds. Add it up: That's more than 115 pounds, from one family member touching the lives of his loved ones.

Without a doubt, *The Biggest Loser* cast members have had a health-building influence wherever they go, including in their own workplaces. Matt's coworkers now look to him for healthy menu suggestions when it's time to order lunch. Whenever there's an office party at the travel agency where Mo Walker works, healthier food selections are served. "My coworkers are really trying to help me maintain my goal and also to eat healthier themselves," Mo said.

If you consider that obesity is associated with more than 30 medical conditions—many of them life-threatening—not only are people like Jeff, Matt, and Mo helping people lose weight, but they're also helping to save precious lives. What greater gift could you give to people than the gift of added years to their lives?

One of the secrets to giving—and receiving—this gift is having and maintaining a strong support system—positive, ongoing contact with other people. You know that if you're trying to lose weight, you're not alone. Weight loss is a goal many people share. People want to lose weight to look better, to feel better, to stay or get healthy, and to live longer. Connecting with them makes the journey so much easier.

Consider the following startling statistic: Approximately 70 percent of dieters who go it alone fail. For many people, these attempts to shed pounds fail because their diets are too rigid and therefore not sustainable, and their approach lacks a support system to help them achieve long-term success.

When you're trying every day to stay the course, you need all the help you can get, including from nondieters. That means telling family, friends, coworkers, and workout partners about your goals and asking for their cooperation. A strong support system should include first and foremost your entire family, and second, a group of friends who can offer camaraderie and encouragement. Every person in your support system can help one another make healthier food choices and begin to exercise. And everyone involved will reap the benefits.

If you don't have a strong support system, or if you'd like some additional backup, check out biggestloserclub.com, an online community of Biggest Losers. Track your weight loss progress, get additional recipes and fitness tips, and share your story with other Biggest Losers.

Lisa Andreone has positive memories of the support element she experienced on the ranch. "Having those other people there, even though they were getting on your nerves at times, was so important. There was so much support and love. Even though we had to eliminate people and that hurt, you could look over at the other cast members and without saying a word, smile at them because you knew they supported you. Seeing them work out on the treadmill and knowing they wanted to lose weight as badly as you did gave you a sense of peace. We were all in this together. The best feeling was knowing you were around people who were as motivated as you were."

Your support system is your cheering section, your fans rooting for you, your chief motivators. Usually, people get really psyched up in the beginning of a fitness program, but in a few weeks, motivation can wane. That's when your support system can keep you going and help you turn your life around.

Once you talk to friends and family about your weight and health goals, you might be surprised to find out that they care more than you know. That's exactly what happened to Jeff Levine. Here's how Jeff described his experience:

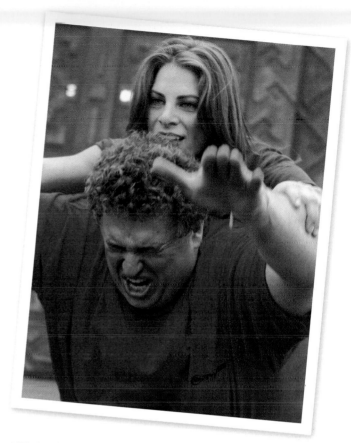

Jeff Levine, during *The Biggest Loser*

• • •

At first I said "no" to The Biggest Loser *— for a lot of reasons. I didn't think it was fair to my wife to leave her with our four kids, all of whom are extremely active. At work, I didn't think my department would let me off. Then I discovered how worried people were about me. My wife had been crying a lot; she feared becoming a widow and having to raise our daughters on her own. My colleagues said they were worried that one day I would drop dead right in the middle of working with a patient. Every single colleague — 28 people — told me that I had to do this. That meant a lot to me, knowing that they would have to work a lot of extra hours to cover for me. Even my patients wanted me to do it. I treat women with a lot of serious physical and emotional problems, and yet many of them started spending most of their time with me, expressing more concern*

about my health than theirs. They'd say, "Dr. Levine, I'm okay; I want to talk about you today. I'm really worried about you; I need you around."

I couldn't believe that my patients, who had all these problems, wanted to spend time asking about my health because they were so concerned about me. I guess because I've always taken care of others, personally and professionally, it was kind of weird that people were more concerned about my health than theirs.

I knew that participating in The Biggest Loser *would be a good thing and that my patients would feel very proud of me for doing it. It's wonderful to know that so many people care about me, support me, and are helping me realize the opportunity to be around for a long time — not only to help my patients, but also to enjoy more time with my family. I am going to be around longer to fight off my daughters' boyfriends. I can actively participate in their lives, whereas before I was becoming a spectator in their lives. My wife and I will have a lot more quality of life as well. That's priceless.*

· · ·

One way you can get in on this priceless gift is to initiate a fun, rather unique form of support right in your own family, workplace, or community: Organize and set up your own Biggest Loser competition.

Think about it: If you walked away from watching *The Biggest Loser* inspired, uplifted, and saying to yourself, "I can do that at home . . . cook like that . . . eat like that . . . exercise like that," and you made the commitment to do it, why not start your own Biggest Loser challenge, in which you and others compete to lose weight through exercise and diet? What do you have to lose — except a lot of weight?

Losing weight with others and throwing in a little friendly competition can be a lot of fun. It will help keep you motivated — even when you don't really feel like it. Everyone wins because everyone who participates and stays with it will lose weight.

Lisa, who made it to the "final five" in season one, is a firm believer in the competitive element of successful weight loss. "If there wasn't a competition, we probably

Important

The Biggest Losers lost lots of weight each week, partly because they were working out several hours each day. The safe and most successful rate of weight loss under normal conditions is 2 pounds per week.

wouldn't have lost as much weight as we did. The first week I lost 15 pounds, and the numbers kept going up. Other than one week where I lost a pound, I always lost 5, 6, or more pounds each week. I've never lost that much weight in a week, in my life. You have so much more motivation when there's competition."

One of the easiest ways to start is with your own coworkers, right in your workplace. After all, that's where you spend most of your waking hours, and encouragement is just a desk or a cubicle away. Research into weight-loss competitions at work supports the idea, too: Organized weight-loss groups in the workplace have a higher success rate than solo dieting does. The group momentum and cohesion give everyone the motivation they need to get serious about losing weight and exercising. It should not be about peer pressure, either; it's about giving lots of support. Most participants end up meeting their weight-loss goals. Not only that, weight-loss competitions boost morale, improve employee relations, and drive down sick days and health care costs. They also tend to keep the work areas free of junk food, which is important. The cast members said that one of their worst temptation times was during the lunch hour at work. Although they'd try to pack healthy lunches for work while dieting, they often succumbed to peer pressure when everyone else ordered pizza or went out for burgers.

Of course, there are lots of other different venues in which you can organize your competition. For example, consider:

- Community
- Neighborhood
- Family
- Friends and social circle
- School/class
- House of worship
- Online community

Keep in mind that it's not just about staging a competition, it's about helping other people try to change their lives and reshape their lifestyles. After you consider where you want to do your Biggest Loser competition and with what group of people, it's time to get organized. Here are the steps to making sure your competition is the best it can be.

Step 1: Consider the timing.

The right timing will help participants stick to their resolutions. After the calorie packed winter holidays, for example, most people are primed to think about fitness because they are starting the new year with a clean slate and a whole year ahead to better themselves. And, as the weather gets warmer, people start thinking about trimming down for the summer—to look good in their bathing suits, at class reunions, for summer trips, and for weddings. That's why January 1 and late spring usually represent good times to get people interested in losing weight. Both are times of renewal, when we're most likely to make lose-weight vows and be motivated to keep them. Of course, feel free to start your challenge any time, especially if you have participants who are gung-ho about it!

Step 2: Recruit contestants.

You'll need to get the word out that you're holding a Biggest Loser competition and set a date for an organizational meeting, in which the rules and guidelines are covered. Here are some avenues to consider for publicity:

- Publicize your Biggest Loser competition by putting the meeting location and time in the community calendar of your local newspaper and radio and television stations.
- Post announcements or inexpensive flyers at doctors' offices, clinics, hospitals, gyms and fitness centers, spas, libraries, community centers, and social service agencies.
- Use word of mouth to reach new participants. Friends, family members, and neighbors can all help you spread the word.
- Send e-mails to people you know who might be interested or who know people who might benefit from participating in the competition.
- Check out biggestloserclub.com and meet contestants online.

The Biggest Loser Weight-Loss Competition
OFFICIAL RULES

1. The weight-loss competition will run for 12 weeks, beginning _____ and ending _____.

2. You should follow the diet and exercise recommendations from *The Biggest Loser* book as closely as possible.

3. You may enter the competition as an individual or as part of a team. Teams can include up to 10 members.

4. Teams can be made up of men and women, women only, or men only.

5. Each team should create a team name and select a team leader to keep track of the team's progress.

6. Private weekly weigh-ins will be held at _____ (time) at _____ (place). Each person will be weighed on the same scale throughout the competitions.

7. The registration fee is _____.

8. Scoring is based on percent (not number of pounds) of body weight lost per individual or per team.

9. Good attendance helps you stay on track toward meeting your weight-loss goal. If you cannot attend a meeting, contact your team leader. If you have _____ unexcused absences in a row, you'll be disqualified from receiving prizes or awards.

The purpose of this contest is to support your efforts to follow a healthy weight-loss diet and exercise program and to establish patterns that you can continue long after the contest is over. It is not intended to promote rapid weight loss.

Please do not enter if you are already at a healthy weight.

Step 3: Establish a weekly weigh-in location and registration fees.

One important aspect of the competition is the weekly weigh-in. Each week, participants must step on the scale to see whether they've lost weight. This weigh-in should be conducted in private by a designated support person—not another contestant. It's best to schedule weigh-ins at the same designated place each week.

Also, establish a registration fee. These funds can be used to create prizes for the team or the individual (or both) who loses the greatest percent of body weight. You can also use the fees to honor a weekly Biggest Loser or a monthly Biggest Loser—the one who has recorded the highest weight loss for that particular period.

Step 4: Write your rules.

For your competition to be successful, you'll need some official rules for everyone to follow. There's a suggested format for your official rules on the opposite page; feel free to change or adapt it to your own needs.

Step 5: Organize weekly support activities.

Not only is your challenge a competition, but it should also provide support activities through the week for participants. As a team, devise ways to provide positive support to each other and to encourage each person's success.

- Get together during the week to encourage the sharing of experiences: What has worked well for each person and why. This is an opportunity for participants to learn new weight-loss skills, plus strategies for trans-

forming their bodies and their lives. Be sure to share ideas for resisting temptation and staying the course. You'll find that every member contributes something. One person will find a new exercise; someone else will bring in a motivational quote, informative article, or a new recipe that the whole group tries. There is always an opportunity for every member to contribute and for every member to benefit from that contribution.

If your competition is organized at work, lunches and coffee breaks are common gathering times, so use them for support meetings.

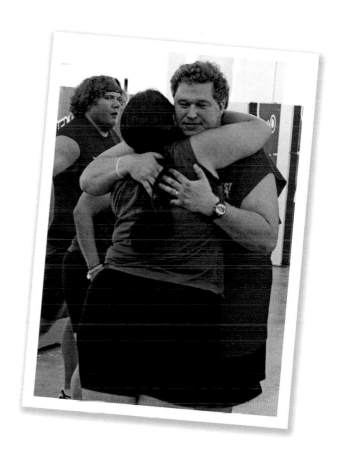

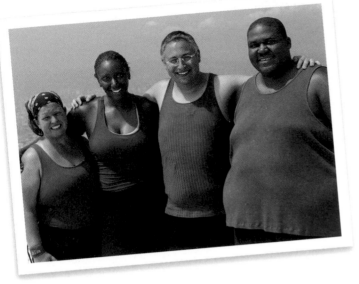

For at least the cost of the instructor, the facility can provide classes in aerobics, yoga, Pilates, and other programs. The advantage is that instructors are usually certified in exercise and safety. Local YMCA branches also allow their facilities to be used as home bases for walking, running, or biking programs. It's certainly worth a phone call.

- Check in with each other to keep each other accountable. Ongoing accountability makes a support group successful. For example, if you're out driving and want to duck into a fast-food restaurant, you can call one of your members who can tell you to stay away. Sometimes it's hard to avoid temptation, but it's not as hard when someone is keeping you accountable. When you're re-

- Join together to walk or to exercise.
- Enter 5Ks or 10Ks together.
- Organize social events or other special activities, such as potluck dinners using Biggest Loser recipes.
- Dine out together in restaurants that offer healthy options in order to practice and apply healthy dining-out strategies.
- Attend health lectures and programs as a group.
- Sign up for a walk-a-thon or other activity-oriented fundraiser as a group. Such activities give you a chance to bond with one another and cement your support for each other.
- Send encouraging e-mails and fitness tips to each other through the week.
- Look into working out a deal with your local YMCA or other fitness facility, which for a fee may help local groups set up exercise programs and provide instructors.

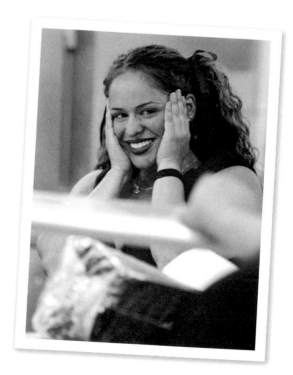

sponsible to another person, it really helps. Knowing that you can check in with someone tomorrow keeps you on track today.

With this kind of support, you have surrounded yourself with a group of people who will encourage you and give you the accountability you need to achieve your goals. There is motivating energy in active, supportive ties to people who want you to do well. With these people in your life, the more likely you and your other members are to succeed.

The benefits of group support transcend weight loss. According to Mo Walker, "I definitely made a lot of friends on the ranch. We were bonded by that common thread of losing weight and getting healthy. I especially plan on staying in touch with Andrea and Gary from my team. Really, I'll keep in touch with just about everybody."

Bottom line: The benefit of the group *is* the group. The group format is always appealing because you're doing it with your friends (new and old), and there's support around you.

Step 6: Create your own Biggest Loser challenges.

Part of the fun of watching *The Biggest Loser* was to see what sort of "challenges" the cast members were put through each week. They pulled cars, ran up the stairs of tall buildings, biked or worked out on the treadmill for hours to see who could rack up the most miles, had relay races on the beach, hauled the weight they had lost in gold bricks, walked on balance beams, and more. You can design similar challenges for your own competition. Here are some ideas to get you started.

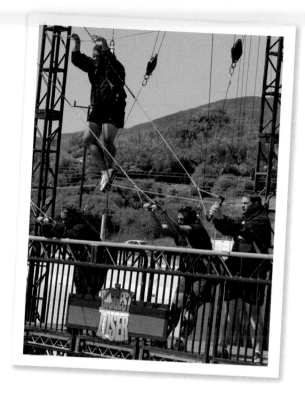

- Have accumulated activity challenges, such as number of hours exercised each week, the number of steps walked (use pedometers), or number of miles walked, run, or biked.
- Set up a spinning class in which you compete to see who can go the farthest in an hour or 90 minutes. Try the same challenge with treadmills.
- Organize a race to see who can climb up the stairs to the top of your office building in the shortest time.
- Have relay races at the city park or your community pool.
- See who can do the most sit-ups or push-ups or jump rope the longest.

- Compete against another Biggest Loser team in a tug-of-war challenge.
- Stage a rock wall climbing contest at a local gym.
- See who can complete a fitness course, with various stations, in the fastest time. Fitness courses, such as Fit-Trails, can be those found in parks, or you can set up your own at a local gym.

Step 7: Celebrate!

It's a great touch to wind up the 12 weeks with a celebration in which awards are handed out. You might consider a team award to the group who brought home the gold, in addition to individual awards. If you held your competition at work, consider having a rotating trophy created for the competition, especially if you decide to make the competition a yearly event at your office.

Prizes should be health-inspired—not a trip to the ice cream parlor, for example! Prize ideas might include:

- Fitness gear such as a gym bag, jogging suit, jump rope or exercise tubing, stability ball, medicine ball, or a set of free weights
- Gift certificate to a sporting goods store
- A massage, facial, manicure, or pedicure at a local salon
- A weekend trip to a health spa
- A free supply of bottled water for 1 year
- A year's membership to a local gym or health club

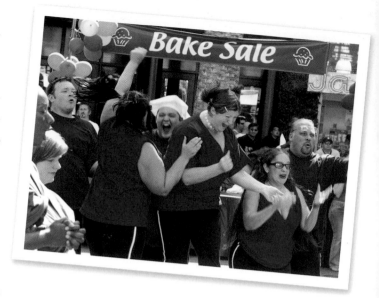

- A piece of cardio equipment such as a treadmill or stationary bicycle
- 10 sessions with a personal trainer
- Cash prizes for the top individual winner and second and third runners-up

Organizing your Biggest Loser competition and getting others involved will net you much more than prizes. Your new trim, healthier body will be reward enough. You and your team members will get closer to your fighting weights, you'll feel good, you'll look great, and you'll most likely add years to your lives. This won't be just a game to you. It will be a life change.

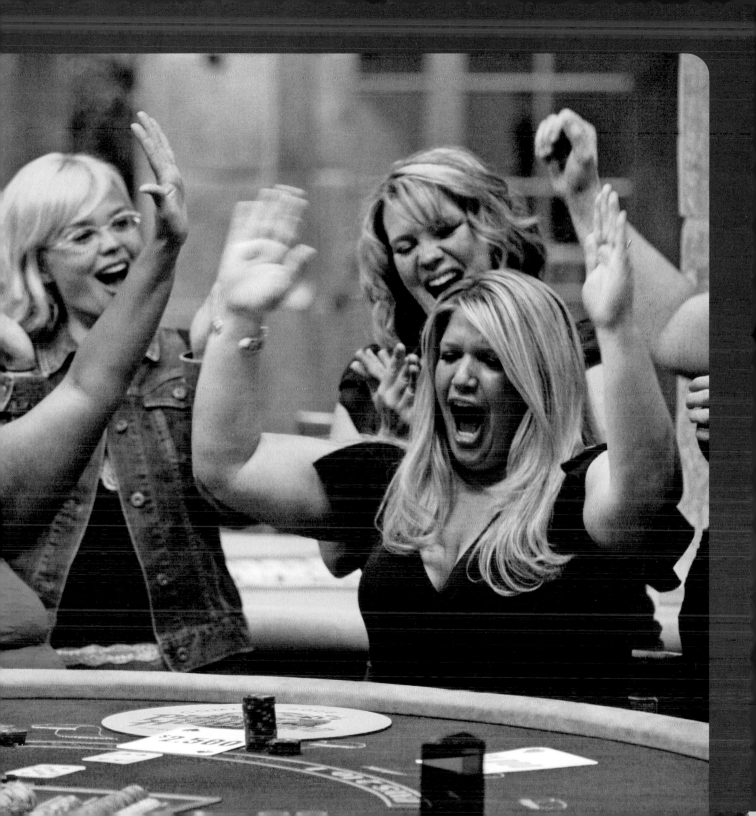

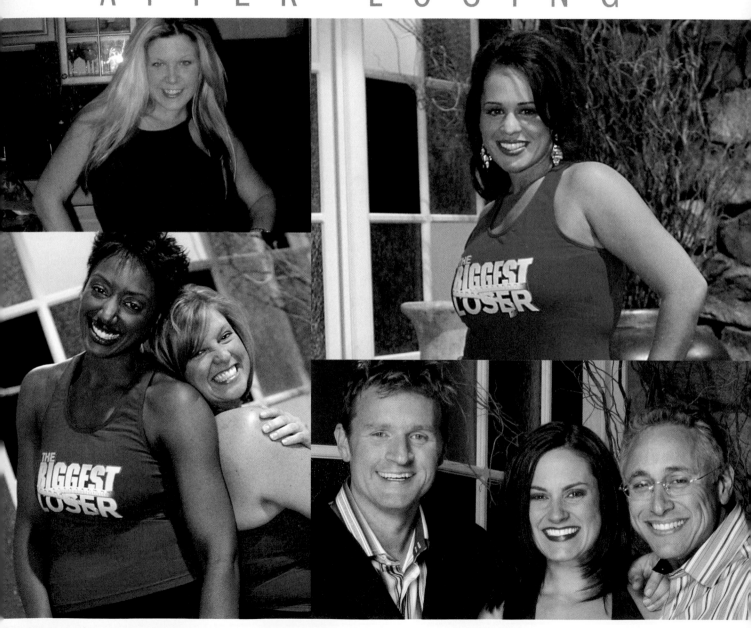

What's more challenging than trying to lose weight? Keeping those pounds off!

Most of the Biggest Losers would agree that they were once your classic yo-yo dieters, with their weight going up and down all the time, never with any long-term success at keeping it off. Dana DeSilvio yo-yoed in a big way, trying four diets in a month at one desperate point. "I started a carb diet, a no-carbs diet, then a shake diet, and finally a low-calorie diet. None involved exercise, and they all failed." Suzy Preston was no different: "I have tried diets all my life. All through high school, I was a yo-yo dieter, too. I was either on a diet or absolutely not on a diet." Like so many people on diets, both women eventually yo-yoed in a big way. Dana hit 175 pounds; Suzy, 227 pounds.

Unfortunately, the statistics on the probability of keeping your weight off are not always the best news: Of those who do successfully lose weight, 90 to 95 percent are unable to keep it off over the long haul. This is worrisome, since being overweight is so intricately linked with so many physical and mental health problems, including heart disease, diabetes, cancer, and depression. While one in three adults is trying to lose weight, another 50 percent are attempting to maintain their current weight, according to the Centers for Disease Control and Prevention (CDC).

Who will succeed? The Biggest Losers provide some important insights for beating the odds.

Stay Diet-Disciplined

The Biggest Losers keep their calories down, consume food and drinks low in fat and sugar, eat smaller-portioned meals, eat natural carbohydrates, incorporate lots of fruits and vegetables, and focus on foods high in fiber. They shun obvious nutritional no-nos such as processed food, white sugar, and excessive alcohol. They know how to make substitutions for higher-calorie foods, such as nonfat, no-sugar ice cream for real ice cream, Wasa bread for bagels, or spaghetti squash for pasta. They also make sure to eat four to six meals a day, spaced about 3 hours apart, in order to curb cravings and keep their metabolisms humming along.

Stay Realistic

It's just not realistic to say that you'll never eat apple pie or cheesecake ever again. There will be times when you will, and you'll feel like a failure when you break your self-imposed "never-eat-this-or-that" rule. It is more realistic, however, to build those calories into your plan or compensate for the additional calories by doing more exercise. Andrea Overstreet said, "I did eat some of my favorite chocolate while on the ranch, but it was okay because I made sure that I still had room for it in my calorie allotment for the day."

Dana DeSilvio agreed. "If I want something like a couple of cookies or an ice cream cone, I will eat it because you just can't cut everything out for the rest of your life. Besides, I'll just work it off the next day."

You must accept the fact that you will be seduced by tempting foods yet realize you can still eat these foods in moderation, so that you won't feel deprived. That's what real-life eating is all about.

When his clients get close to their goal weights, trainer Bob Harper often advises them to take 1 day a week to eat whatever they like, such as chips or some candy. A few of the Biggest Losers such as Ryan Benson have chosen to incorporate this advice into their plan, while others like Gary Deckman prefer to stay consistent with the eating plan. It all depends on what you think will work best for you. A free day or a free meal simply means that you eat whatever you want and forget about calories, carbs, or fat for a day or for a meal.

Having one free day of eating or having one free meal once in a while probably won't sabotage your ability to control your weight, yet you shouldn't make a habit of it. If you find that free days or free meals are a problem for you and too much of a temptation, then don't include them in your maintenance plan. Simply find a way to include an occasional treat without overindulging. As Bob puts it, "Losing weight and keeping it off means balance, not going without treats for the rest of your life."

Stay Active

A national survey conducted by the Calorie Control Council asked people who said they need to lose weight why they hadn't been successful at maintaining their desired weight. The number one answer: "Don't exercise enough." Clearly, not staying active keeps many a loser from winning the maintenance game!

That's why, in addition to monitoring their diet, the Biggest Losers still engage in high levels of activity to remain trim—and they do so on a regular basis. They report exercising anywhere from three to six times a week, usually for an hour or an hour and a half each workout. On the advice of *The Biggest Loser* trainers, Bob and Jillian, the cast members keep their bodies guessing by doing a variety of exercises and workouts.

Ryan Benson's exercise program includes mountain biking, for example. "I usually ride three mornings a week for 90 minutes; then I attend spin classes at the gym 2 days a week. I also do some weight training twice a week for good measure."

Suzanne Mendonca works out twice a day—in the morning and again at night. Her workouts include spinning classes, working out on an elliptical trainer, and running anywhere from 4 to 6 miles a day.

Lisa Andreone meets with her trainer three times a week for weight training and does about an hour of cardio afterward. "On the days I am not with my trainer, I go to a Latin cardio and dance class. Both are great for the body."

Although they rely mostly on cardio exercise to stay in shape, their activities include weight training, spin classes, dancing, yoga, Pilates, boot camp classes, hiking, kickboxing, various sports, and more. They burn an average of 1,500 to 4,500 calories per week each, which is a surefire formula for successful weight loss and maintenance.

A growing body of research suggests that weight training helps keep pounds off, which is why the cast members include this form of exercise in their fitness programs. While cardio burns the fat, weight training creates shape and develops lean muscle. With body-firming muscle, your metabolism runs faster, even while you're at rest. Weight training is a must for weight management and maintenance.

Stay Accountable

As mentioned earlier, successful weight-loss maintenance seems to require consistent "self-monitoring." For instance, some of the Biggest Losers weigh themselves daily, some weekly, while others keep an accurate food journal, write down meal plans, or keep their "fat pictures" in plain view. If the scale creeps up a bit, they know what to do—cut back on calories, processed carbs, or fat or exercise a little more.

Continue to keep your food journal, even through maintenance. A food journal can help you identify your motives for overeating, whether they involve stress, emotions, fatigue, boredom, or certain places or social situations. You can write down not only what you eat, but also why you eat. Writing this information down brings it into the light and helps you analyze it, so that you can avoid the situation in the future. You'll know that the next time you have a run-in with your boss or boyfriend and you want to stuff yourself with a box of cookies, you can stop off at the gym instead and sweat off your frustration.

In short, self-monitoring techniques are important reminders of what you're doing and can inspire you to keep going.

Their Winning Ways

Despite the differing techniques they use to manage their weight and keep it off, the Biggest Losers do agree on what is necessary to win: They all say it takes long-term lifestyle changes, not short-term crash diets. You are more likely to keep your weight off with pound-paring lifestyle changes such as eating more wholesome foods, lowering your caloric and fat intake, and exercising. If you lose weight by changing your lifestyle, then keeping the weight off will be less work. Thinking positively about your lifestyle changes—that you're doing this for your health, your family, and your future—can make it easier to keep that weight off, too.

While making lifelong behavioral changes can be daunting, there is some reassuring news: Research shows that people who have maintained their weight loss for 3 to 5 years say that it gets easier, as long as you continue the good eating and exercise habits you developed while losing weight.

Every one of the 12 contestants on season one managed to lose a lot of weight during the show. Better yet: They also all managed to keep losing after leaving the ranch. The Biggest Losers showed America that it is possible to go back into their lives and to survive and thrive with what they learned during their experience. In their own words, here is how they celebrate life after losing.

Lisa Andreone

When I first got to the ranch, I weighed a ridiculous 236 pounds. I wasn't living a healthy lifestyle. I could have died at a young age. By the time I left the ranch, I had gotten down to 189, which makes it 47 pounds in total. After I got home, I kept up my diet, I kept up my exercise, I got a personal trainer, and now I've lost an additional 20 pounds, making my total weight loss 67 pounds. I've adapted everything in my life around exercising and eating right. Both are a part of my life. I feel like I saved myself, and I got out of my rut.

It feels wonderful to be thinner. I barely used to squeeze into a 16, but now I'm just sliding into a 10, and I love it. I

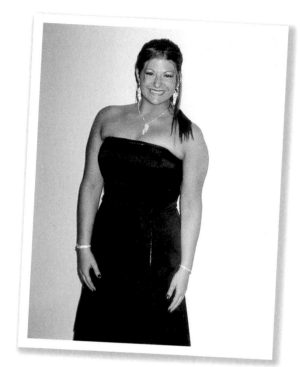

Lisa Andreone, after *The Biggest Loser*

can wear whatever I want. I can show off my arms. I feel confident.

Being on *The Biggest Loser* totally transformed my lifestyle. I am not the old Lisa who first came to that ranch—crabby, whiny, and humongous. Now I'm always smiling, laughing, and joking. I just feel so good about myself. I am such a better person now than I was back then—more positive, outgoing, and confident.

The game may be over on the ranch, but I feel like the game has just started for my life. I love to go dancing now, for example. It's something I live for. I have more energy. I can last longer on the dance floor. I'm not worried about pulling down my shirt to cover up a chubby roll. I just feel so free. I can wear my sexy shoes and sexy clothes and just go. I can let loose, dance with my friends, and not worry about what my arms look like. I just love to tear it up and let loose. I love dancing now more than ever.

This has been a lifestyle change, not only physically, but emotionally. I used to be a very negative person, and I basically had to go through a transformation to become what I am right now.

Andrea ("Drea") Baptiste

Things are great. I'm back hard at work doing sales and making the time to eat right and work out. I still manage

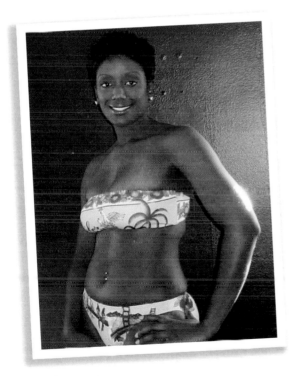

Drea Baptiste, after *The Biggest Loser*

to meet people on the street who ask for advice, and I'm happy to share.

When I first got to the ranch, I weighed a whopping 215 pounds and wore a size 16. It's still hard to say those numbers. Today, I am 164 pounds, for a total weight loss of about 51 pounds.

When I walk out of a dressing room with a size 6 on, I feel like a runway model, and I'm the star of the fashion show. I feel like I'm strutting on the catwalk, down to the mirror, doing my twirls and my turns. I enjoy looking at myself in a three-way mirror now, especially wearing something that's strapless because I love my arms. My body is so contoured, too. I can fit into a pair of 100 percent denim, nonstretch jeans, boot cut and low rise. I can also wear a bikini—a dream of mine.

Dressed to go to a club, I look at myself, and say, "Wow, you did that. You put that outfit on. You put on your little miniskirt and your high heel shoes. Girl, you go out and rock them." I can't even tell you how ecstatic I am every day to get dressed. Every day is a great day. I like what I see.

I feel like a superhighway, too. My body's just going, burning, enjoying the exercise, enjoying the good food, and getting great results.

Losing this weight has been by far the most rewarding opportunity of a lifetime. I don't see anything that could possibly beat this in my past, and I don't foresee anything possibly coming close to this in my future, because this experience has been a complete inside out change. I feel like the caterpillar who went into its cocoon for a period of time, then came out as a beautiful butterfly. That's my transformation, coming out into the world and feeling free to soar in every way possible.

Ryan Benson

Since being crowned the Biggest Loser on season one, there is nothing I love to hear more than "Hey, aren't you *The Biggest Loser* guy?" Being a "Big Loser" is a title I wear with pride! I really worked myself to the bone the week before the final weigh-in. I gave myself a couple of weeks off after that, but I noticed that I was really craving the workouts (I also noticed the weight was creeping back on!). My

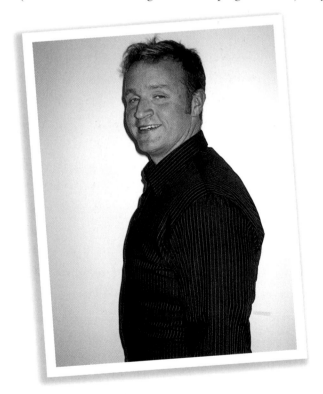

Ryan Benson, after *The Biggest Loser*

starting weight at the ranch was 330, and I've lost more than 100 pounds.

This Saturday, I went surfing for the first time in 3 years, and it was amazing. I just cruised through the water while paddling, and I was able to just pop up on the board. There were probably 200 surfers out there that day in Manhattan Beach. I'll bet I was the happiest guy there because I didn't get tired.

I went to a play recently and unlike other times, I did not have to find a seat in the aisle. I could sit anywhere and not feel cramped. Also, I can go in any store and buy the clothes I want.

Almost every day, someone says to me, "You look so good." That's nice to hear. I'd be lying if I said I didn't enjoy that aspect of it.

My wife, Mariah, and I recently took a trip to Yosemite to go hiking. This was great, not only for my health, but also for my marriage because it brought my wife and me closer together. It was good for me emotionally and good for me spiritually. Being lighter makes me a happier person, and when I'm happier, I'm a better husband.

Even on Christmas morning, I did something I thought I'd never do in a million years: Mariah and I opened our presents and then went out jogging for an hour.

My biggest accomplishment since beginning this journey has been sticking to it. My diet and exercise routine are definitely a new way of living for me. I've never stuck to anything this long in my life. Staying with it has proved to me that I can accomplish whatever I set out to do.

The best thing I've been doing since the show ended is working to help get kids as healthy as possible. I've been speaking at elementary schools teaching kids about how important it is to live a healthy lifestyle. I know from growing up overweight how tough it can be for kids these days, so hopefully I can help show them the benefits of a healthy lifestyle. I am also working on producing and hosting a daily show for kids that would promote kid-appropriate exercise, healthy eating ideas, and an all-around fun and healthy life.

I plan more life changes ahead. Mariah and I want to start our own family as soon as possible. That's one reason I wanted to get fit: to be there for our kids.

Lizzeth Davalos

Since the show, I've been working hard, keeping my weight at 145 pounds, but I didn't stop there! I work out four times a week, run 5 miles a day with my dog, and stick to a very strict diet: no more cheating! It's best to take life day by day, and I am keeping at this, making sure I'm doing everything the right way.

The show really developed my sense of self-worth and helped me avoid trying to take the easy way out, as I have in my past. Now is the time to do it, and I don't want to get to 40 years old without ever having worn a two-piece swimsuit. I'm excited for the summers and especially looking forward to going to the beach. I've felt better than I ever have in my life, and I am really trying to get the rest of my family to get into better shape as well, helping them make better choices with their food and teaching them how to exercise. I keep telling them: "Don't wait until Monday, start today!"

I never stopped living what I learned on the ranch. The habits I learned are things I can do for the rest of my life. I am so committed to staying in shape and being healthy. I want to be around for as long as I can.

My advice to overweight people in America is to stick to it. Don't give up. Even if you fail once, try again. Even if you fail twice, try again. Even if you have tried dozens and dozens of times, try again. You've just got to stay focused and put your heart into it.

Gary Deckman

First, let me just tell you that I'm not feeling good, I'm feeling great! Sure, I didn't win the $250,000, but I did win a new life. I started the show weighing 227, which is not really all that big, but my body fat percentage was 36 percent. I have toned up and am tipping the scales at a cool 160, with around 10 to 11 percent body fat, which is good for me. I feel very strong. I'm very healthy. I'm confident that I can stay on this plan indefinitely. This is the way I will live my life from now on.

When I was overweight, I could barely run around the block. Now I'm running 3 to 5 miles a day. At 40 years old, I've completed a 10K race, so I know I can run 6.2 miles at once. It made me feel great because I never thought I could run that far . . . ever! But I finished it, and I could have kept going!

I know that if I go into something with a losing attitude, I'm already setting myself up for failure. But if I go in with a winning attitude, meaning that I'll succeed, then I will. My trainer on the ranch, Bob Harper, gave me some invaluable advice: "When Michael Phelps is in the pool swimming,

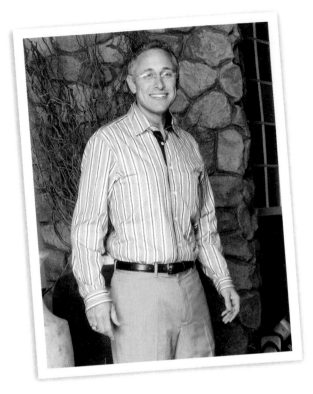

Gary Deckman, after *The Biggest Loser*

what is he thinking about? He's thinking about one thing, and that's swimming faster. When Lance Armstrong is in a race, what is he thinking about? Pedaling faster." That's what I'm relying on and remembering: staying consistent, running faster, and winning.

Things with my wife and kids are great. Our weekends are usually filled with bike trips along the beach and hikes in the Malibu Mountains. My wife looks at me like she did when we were both 18 years old. That's after 23 years of being together. Every night, she's waiting at the door, wondering when I'm going to get home, just to see me. After more than 2 decades of being together, she's still excited to

see me, now more than ever. That's such an uplifting thing for me. I don't want that to ever stop.

Losing weight and getting healthier has been a renewal for me. I've gained a whole new outlook.

Dana DeSilvio

I'm still losing weight and "getting 'er done," as I like to say. I started at 175 and am now down to 147. I have every intention of making every head turn, as I get leaner; in fact, I hope they break their necks!

I came home from the ranch with a new eating style, a new exercising style, and just a new lifestyle. Mostly what I have been watching is my sugar, and that's working for me. I keep everything with only 1 or 2 grams of sugar or sugar-free. As for the rest of the food, I love grilled chicken, salad, celery, broccoli, cauliflower, and raw vegetables. I love it all.

Usually, I work out three or four times a week for about 2 hours a day, which is really helping my metabolism. I'm starting to like a lot more of my body parts. My arms are getting a lot more defined, and my calves are hot. My legs look great, too. I'm really concentrating on my stomach, because that's my problem area. But the rest of me is getting really toned, and I'm really excited about how I look and feel.

These days, I'm a team leader for MSN.com's Losing Weight with Family. I'm going to be in a bathing suit competition for Planet Beach (a tanning company). I just got a house with my new boyfriend in Kentucky and, boy, do I love the country. I'm happy about the new Dana, but basically, I'm still the same country lovin' girl. Like I always say, "Save a horse, ride a cowboy!"

I'm very proud of myself for doing all this, and I feel great about it. It feels so good to hear people say that I look better. I'm just so happy that I've completely turned my life around and I'm headed toward a better life.

I tell people all the time that no one is going to get you to lose weight, you have to do it yourself. You can do it because it is possible. I mean, look at what we 12 people did!

Dave Fioravanti

When I came home from the ranch, I took my fitness goals very seriously because I wanted to prove that I shouldn't have been voted off. I set my sights on winning the $100,000 consolation prize and beating out the other eight eliminated contestants on the reunion show—and I did. But the real payoff has been looking and feeling great. I gave myself 2 weeks off after that victory. Then I realized that I really liked eating healthy and working out, so I jumped back into my new healthy lifestyle.

Core fusion classes (Pilates, aerobics, yoga, and dance) in conjunction with weight lifting and cardio are my thing now. As far as my diet goes, I still basically eat clean good food and watch my calories. My idea of cheating now is a huge bowl of low-carb cereal with fruit. People stop me in the street all the time to tell me how I have inspired them, and I like that. I like making people feel good! When you feel good, you look good.

Before *The Biggest Loser,* I was nearly 260 pounds; now I'm weighing in at a toned 183. I came away from the show with a metamorphosis to a better Dave. I like the way I feel. I like the way I look. I like myself in my clothes. I like buttoning my jeans and not having to suck my stomach in to get them buttoned.

Most people don't realize the extent to which the show changed my life. I used to be the guy who was out until 4:00 in the morning every night, partying and drinking heavily. For me, the show was like rehab. In one day, I had to give up not only a lot of foods, but also alcohol and cigarettes. I'm not that unhealthy guy anymore. What keeps me going now is how great I feel. I never want to return to that old Dave.

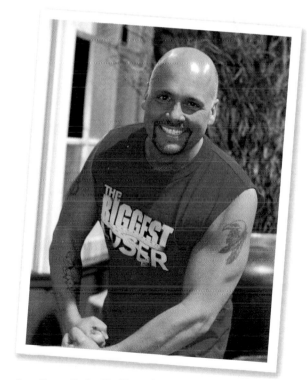

Dave Fioravanti, after *The Biggest Loser*

Matt Kamont

I'm living fabulous! I started at 310 and am now dancing on the scale at 240 pounds. A 70-pound loss! I'm working on losing more weight. Basically, I have cut out processed carbs, and I eat lots of salad, chicken, and fruit. I don't do fast food, really. That isn't even in my vocabulary. The biggest take-home message I learned from my experience at the ranch is that fad diets do not work.

Portion control is a new way of life for me. Instead of having half a container, I have a small mug of ice cream. I'm less of an emotional eater, thanks to keeping a food journal, but I'm still an emotional person. I work out three times a week for an hour a day. I do 100 push-ups on the stairs and sit-ups every night! If you think I started smoking again, guess again!

I've been asked to teach a fitness class at the gym where I work out. It's a class that will teach people the techniques I learned at the ranch, so I'm in the process of planning that. I can't wait to start watching people's weight diminish!

Friends and family have been inspired and many are losing weight and that makes me feel good. My advice to those interested: Take the stairs, park far away, and live fabulous!

Kelly MacFarland

I feel jacked up. When I first arrived at the ranch, I was 223 pounds; now I weigh 154 pounds. I work out like a fiend—1 hour a day, 6 days a week—see a trainer twice a week, and still keep a food journal. I've found a determination I never even knew had existed.

Exercise is my key. It allows me to eat dessert and frozen yogurt. I had real ice cream once but felt weird about it. My parents are working out now, and my roommate has lost more than 25 pounds.

I'm going on dates. Yes, I actually get asked for my digits these days! I consider being on *The Biggest Loser* just a monumental experience. I'm a different person, and I like me.

My experience has been a complete physical and mental makeover. I call it a "soul makeover."

Kelly Minner

Since *The Biggest Loser* finale, I am back at school and really excited to be working with my students again in a creative way. They are a daily reminder to me of why I did this, and they keep me on the right track. One of the reasons I did the show was to pass on a legacy to let these kids know that, yes, dreams do come true. Every day that I see their worth and potential, I realize my own.

I have kids who are coming up to me and saying, "Miss Minner, you inspired me to lose weight." Then they do it and get fit. This is so rewarding to see! Their parents have told me, "You can't imagine what you've done for my child. Thank you!"

I have stayed on track because for the first time in my life I found I am worth it and I am not giving that up. I'm toned, and gosh, stronger and happier and healthier, and that feels so good. What I can wear now has changed, too. Now I can put on low-rise pants. Jackets now fit me because my arms are more slender. I used to be scared to look at myself in a

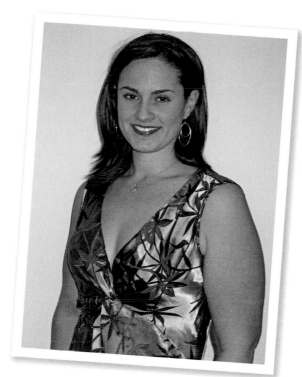

Kelly Minner, after *The Biggest Loser*

Aaron Semmel

Life is good. Before I came on the show, I weighed in at 261 pounds. Now I'm down to 199. I'm at 11 percent body fat now, and I'm still working toward my goal of being down to 6 percent body fat.

I took a couple weeks off after the reunion show, but now I'm training hard again, and I feel fantastic. For me, it's all about exercise.

I wake up every day and start my day with like a mile swim and at least an hour in the gym. I also do a circuit-training routine, like we learned at the ranch. I need to build

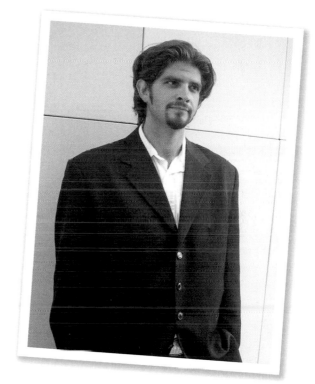

Aaron Semmel, after *The Biggest Loser*

mirror. Not anymore. What's looking back at me in that mirror makes me so happy.

My life has changed so immensely. I'm a different person. I'm a calmer person. Whereas I used to have this manic energy, now I have a serenity that I want to carry with me forever.

I've learned how to be nice to myself, too. I often go home and treat myself to a bubble bath or a pedicure—any reward as long as it's not food. I've worked too hard now to fail at this! I have new habits that I fully intend to keep. This has been a lifestyle change, and it has given me a new life.

The Cast Members' Best Tips for Maintenance

- Stay aware of what you're eating and how many calories your food contains.
- Eat four to six meals a day to enhance your metabolism.
- Choose low-fat, low-calorie, and low-carb versions of your favorite foods.
- Enjoy your meals, savor each bite, and eat more slowly, rather than wolfing them down.
- Eat plenty of fruits and vegetables.
- Learn to love spaghetti squash as a pasta substitute. We all do!
- Pay attention to portion control.
- Plan ahead and prepare your meals ahead of time.
- Don't give into stress eating; if you feel like medicating yourself with food, do something else such as exercising, reading, meditating, walking your dog, or treating yourself to a facial or manicure.
- Deal effectively with emotional overeating by telling yourself over and over again that you are in control of your life.
- Limit the amount of alcohol you drink.
- Let yourself have a small amount of a treat, without eating too much of it.
- Monitor your weight on a regular basis. Give yourself a 3- to 5-pound weight gain range that you will not go over. If you exceed it, get back on your program at once.
- Make a list of all the reasons why you do not want to regain your weight.
- Don't spend too much time moping around about a setback or it will be too hard to get remotivated. Get back on your program the next day, the next meal, or the next workout.
- Exercise, exercise, exercise.
- Remember who is the most important person in your life: you!

up my muscles because your muscles are what burn your fat, and right now I'm to the point where I have only small pockets of fat on my body. I've literally melted away most of the fat.

All of these activities give me the energy literally to just crank through the entire day. These are all the things I wanted to do, not because I'm an athlete but because I just love doing them. Like for me, I was fat in high school and I would run in gym class and hate it. Then when I got older, all of the sudden, I fell in love with running. Unfortunately, I got fat again and I couldn't do it.

Since leaving the show, I've done a triathlon. I've climbed to the top of a very tall building, too. I just lead a totally active life.

Things with my girlfriend, Sarah, are still going strong. I jog to her house, and that's 3 miles away! She thinks my new body is fun and nice. She's never known me this skinny. She has always known me at a big, hefty 250. I'll take off my shirt sometimes, and she'll literally see a new muscle.

I've started writing a book about my weight-loss experience, which is cool because it really makes me get inside my own head and it also keeps me motivated.

I've always had a high level of self-confidence, but accomplishing a fitter body and better health has taught me that if you work hard enough, you can do anything.

Maurice ("Mo") Walker

Let me tell you something: The man formerly known as the "overweight Southern lover" has never gotten so much attention from the ladies as he is getting now! I'm making appearances on *The Southern Woman Show* in a special segment called "Cooking MoLicious Style." I beat out Oprah Winfrey to be the Tennessee spokesperson for the Department of Health.

When I showed up at *The Biggest Loser,* I was 436 pounds, and I was on a death sentence, basically. At the ranch, I lost 56 pounds. Since the Reunion Weigh-In, I have lost more weight, bringing me down to 351. I would like to get down to 235, and I think that goal is attainable.

I have a whole new outlook on nutrition and exercise. I don't eat the same foods that I used to eat. Yes, I'm still a Southern boy, but now I eat healthy Southern cooking. In regard to my diet, I'm eating six smaller meals a day, which helps me keep up my metabolism and keep up with the ladies. Mama has reformed her cooking and now bakes chicken as opposed to frying it.

The Biggest, Healthiest Losers

Not only does shedding pounds make you look and feel great, it's one of the best moves you can make for your health. You can significantly reduce your risk of life-shortening illnesses, and as a result, experience everything life has to offer. As proof, here's what several of the Biggest Losers from seasons one and two discovered about how losing weight won back their health.

Jeff Levine. Jeff arrived at the ranch at a hefty 370 pounds. At that point, his blood pressure was soaring at around 160/90, considered seriously high. Now it's back down in a normal range. He has not had to wear his sleep apnea mask since starting the Biggest Loser diet and exercise program. Jeff feels like he looks 10 years younger.

Peter Thomas. Peter arrived at the ranch tipping the scales at 407 pounds. His blood pressure was 150/90, considered high. In just 1 week of following the Biggest Loser diet and exercise program, his blood pressure dropped to a healthy 102/60.

Lisa Andreone. When she was overweight, Lisa suffered from a painful condition called irritable bowel syndrome (IBS), characterized by a group of symptoms in which abdominal pain or discomfort is associated with a change in bowel pattern, such as loose or more frequent bowel movements, diarrhea, and/or constipation. But after she lost a total of 67 pounds, the symptoms subsided, and she no longer takes medication. Her doctor told her: "You're fine. No medicine could have helped you better than losing weight did."

Gary Deckman. Prior to being on *The Biggest Loser,* Gary was on cholesterol-lowering medication, heartburn medicine, and asthma medicine. He is off almost all his medicines now and is taking much lower doses of his asthma medicine.

Suzanne Mendonca. After having her medical examination as part of being a cast member, Suzanne was shocked to learn that her total cholesterol was 265. Within the first 2 weeks, it dropped to 177—a change she calls "amazing."

Dave Fioravanti. When he arrived at the ranch, Dave's cholesterol number was about as high as his weight: 260. After he lost 71 pounds, that number dropped to a healthy 160, all without medication. In fact, one physician wanted to know what kind of cholesterol medication he was taking. Dave told him, "None!" The physician said, "That's impossible!" Dave also reported that he had chronic back pain when he started the show, but the pain vanished after the 4th day of exercising at the ranch. "My health is great because of being on *The Biggest Loser.*"

My idea of exercising before *The Biggest Loser* was walking to the store for food. Now my idea of exercising is jogging past the store. I work out 5 days a week in the gym for an hour and a half, and I also find myself taking the stairs and the long way around in parking lots. Whereas on the ranch, I started out walking a 2.2 mph on the treadmill, today I'm running a 6 mph speed—almost 3 times as fast as when I first got to the ranch.

I feel wonderful in the morning. I feel wonderful when I go to sleep at night. I even feel wonderful after working out. Now that's a big change for me.

I coach a kids' football team. Before, I couldn't even run or exercise with them. Now I can. I can just see on the kids' faces that they appreciate Coach Walker even more.

I've changed my life. It's a whole new Mo. Not only have I lost weight, I've gotten healthier. My blood pressure and my cholesterol, for example, have come way down, and I truly feel good about myself now.

I've been described as being "morbidly obese," and I know there are millions of Americans out there who are morbidly obese, too. I want them to know that if I can do it, they can do it. What's more, I want to show people like me there are other options besides gastric bypass surgery. I want them to gain strength from what I've done. If I can change just one person's life, it's definitely all worth it.

I have a long way to go, but America, you better watch out. Mo is on the way.

Now It's Your Turn

These stories are true reminders of the importance and power of vibrant physical and mental health—of doing everything you can to get fit and in shape. There is something incredible about feeling as good as you can. That feeling is attainable, but it does take work and discipline.

The way to make this happen for yourself is to follow the examples of the Biggest Losers. You can start by trying the eating and exercise plans in this book, and finding a beginner exercise class or a trainer to teach you the ropes. Talk to your doctor about your health; learn what you can improve with some basic lifestyle changes. Make your quest to get in shape a family affair, too. Reread this book often enough so that it continues to fuel your inspiration. Begin to experience how small lifestyle changes can enhance your feelings of well-being and happiness.

What have you got to lose?

Absolutely nothing—except an unhealthy lifestyle that can compromise your health, happiness, and quality of life.

A healthier weight can be yours. And that's just for starters. As the cast members discovered, you'll have more energy, you'll look and feel younger, you'll be more confident, and you'll be better protected against disease.

How great is that?

When you're a biggest loser, too, changing your life and reshaping your lifestyle, you become the biggest winner in the end.

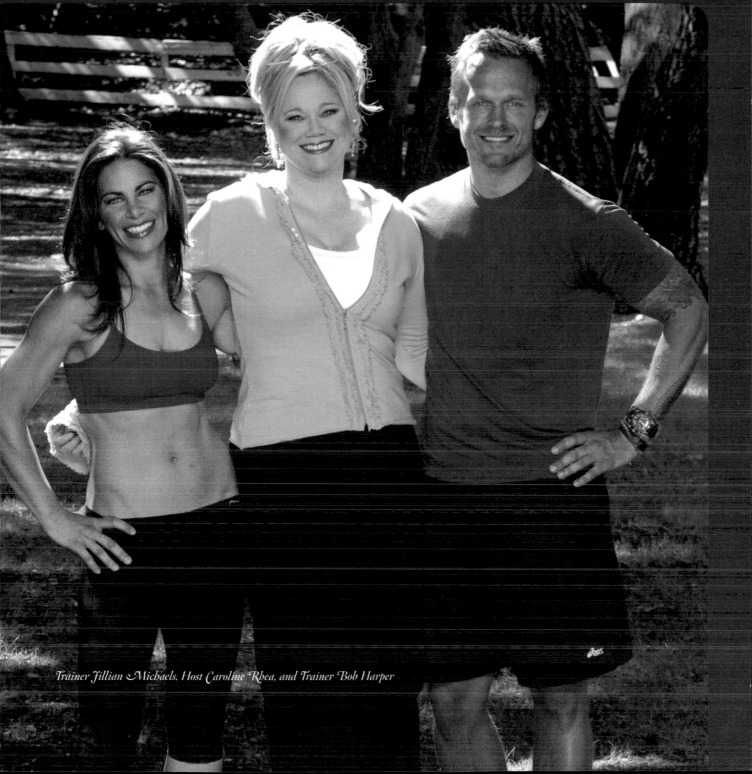

Trainer Jillian Michaels, Host Caroline Rhea, and Trainer Bob Harper

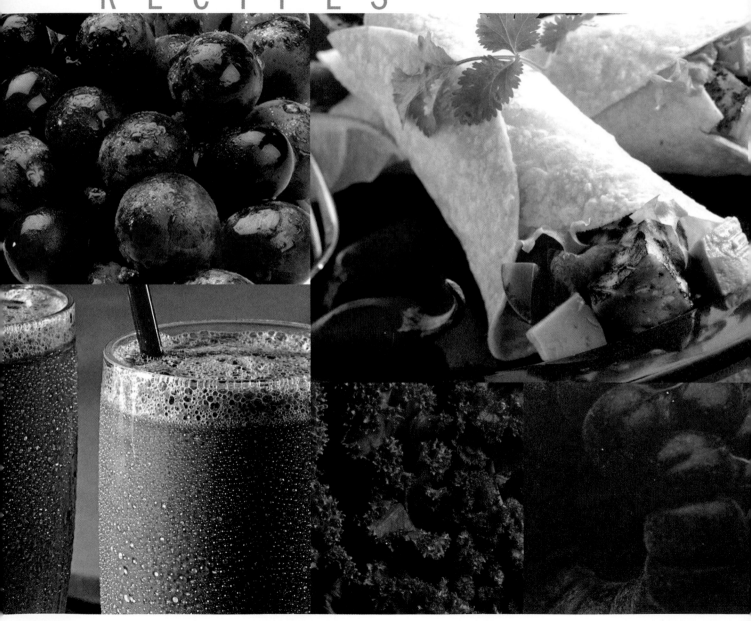

8 The Biggest Loser

RECIPES

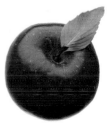

breakfast

SPICY BREAKFAST GRAINS
Yield: 3 cups; 6 (½-cup) servings

A whisper of sweet spices results in complex flavors and a stunningly simple breakfast treat.

1	**teaspoon olive oil**
1	**cup coarse grind bulgur**
1½	**teaspoons fennel seeds**
2	**cups water**
1	**teaspoon vanilla extract**
½	**teaspoon ground cardamom**
½	**teaspoon ground cinnamon**
	Pinch nutmeg
1	**cup blueberries or other fresh berries**

Heat the oil in a 2-quart saucepan over medium heat. Add the bulgur and fennel seeds and cook, stirring frequently, until the bulgur is light golden brown, about 5 minutes. Remove the saucepan from the heat. Carefully stir in the water, vanilla, cardamom, cinnamon, and nutmeg. Return to the heat and bring to a boil. Reduce heat to low, cover, and simmer until most, but not all, of the liquid has been absorbed, about 8 minutes. Remove from heat and allow to stand for 2 minutes.

Spoon into serving dishes. Garnish with blueberries and serve.

Bulgur Factoid: Bulgur is made by boiling whole wheat berries, which are then roasted and ground to the desired texture. Because it is precooked, bulgur is relatively quick to prepare.

Nutrient Analysis per serving
100 calories; 3 g protein; 22 g carbohydrates; less than 1 g total fat; 0 g saturated fat; 0 g polyunsaturated fat; 0 g monounsaturated fat; 0 mg cholesterol; 6 g fiber; 6 mg sodium

BANANA FUDGE SMOOTHIE

Yield: 3 cups; four (¾-cup) servings

Creamy and delicious, this smoothie is great for breakfast or a midday pick-me-up. Pour leftover servings into small plastic bags and freeze. When ready to serve, thaw a frozen portion slightly and remix in the blender.

1½   **cups very cold nonfat milk or soymilk**

½   **cup soft silken tofu**

2   **ripe medium bananas, frozen and cut into 1-inch chunks**

2   **tablespoons unsweetened natural cocoa powder**

1   **teaspoon agave nectar or honey**

½   **teaspoon pure vanilla extract**

Combine all ingredients in a blender or food processor. Blend until smooth. Pour into glasses and serve immediately.

Soy Factoid: Soy protein is easier for the kidneys to process than animal protein. This may reduce the risk of certain kidney problems.

Nutrient Analysis per serving
121 calories; 5 g protein; 23 g carbohydrates; less than 1 g total fat; 0 g saturated fat; 0 g polyunsaturated fat; less than 1 g monounsaturated fat; 0 mg cholesterol; 2 g fiber; 44 mg sodium

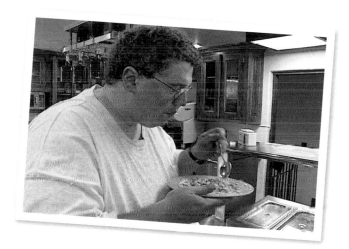

COUNTRY-STYLE TURKEY LINKS

Yield: 16 links; eight 2-link servings

The aroma of these fragrant sausages will lure any sleepyhead to the kitchen. But they're not just for breakfast. They're perfect for a barbecue or crumbled on top of Ryan Benson's Portobello "Pizzas" (see page 136).

1¼ **pounds lean ground turkey (or chicken)**

1 **cup finely chopped leeks (or finely chopped onions)**

½ **cup finely chopped sun-dried tomatoes**

2 **tablespoons chopped fresh basil or parsley**

1 **tablespoon chopped garlic**

2 **teaspoons chopped fresh thyme (or ½ teaspoon dried)**

1 **teaspoon toasted fennel seeds (see note)**

½ **teaspoon freshly ground black pepper**

1 **tablespoon olive oil**

Place all ingredients, except the oil, in the bowl of a food processor. Pulse just until the mixture is well combined and cohesive. Transfer the mixture to a bowl, cover with plastic wrap, and transfer to the freezer for 40 minutes, or until the mixture is very cold, but not frozen. There will be almost 4 cups of mixture. Using slightly less than ¼ cup, quickly shape the mixture into 16 links, each about 3 inches long and 1 inch in diameter (or patties about 2½ inches in diameter).

Heat the oil in a large nonstick sauté pan and brown the sausages over medium heat, turning occasionally, for about 3 minutes. Reduce heat to medium low, cover the pan, and cook, turning the sausages occasionally, until they are crisp and cooked through, about 4 minutes longer. (You may have to do this in two batches.) Drain on paper towels. Serve immediately.

Note: Place fennel seeds in a small sauté pan over medium heat. Toast seeds, stirring occasionally, until fragrant, about 2 minutes. Set aside to cool.

Garlic Factoid: We don't understand the mechanism of all of garlic's healing powers, but it appears to enhance our immune system in a way that fights cancer cells.

Nutrient Analysis per serving
139 calories; 16 g protein; 4 g carbohydrates; 7 g total fat; 3 g saturated fat; less than 1 g polyunsaturated fat; 2 g monounsaturated fat; 51 mg cholesterol; 1 g fiber; 57 mg sodium

BLUEBERRY BRAN MINI MUFFINS

Yield: 24 miniature muffins

Yes, you can still have a muffin for breakfast—but it won't be the size of a grapefruit! Savor blueberries' healthy benefits in moist, delicious mini muffins. They are loaded with fiber and freeze well, too.

1½ **cups unprocessed wheat bran or oat bran**

1 **cup whole wheat flour**

2 **tablespoons ground flaxseed**

1¼ **teaspoons baking soda**

1 **teaspoon ground cinnamon**

⅛ **teaspoon salt**

¾ **cup 1 percent milk or unflavored soymilk**

⅓ **cup honey**

1 **ripe medium banana, mashed with a fork**

1 **large egg**

2 **tablespoons olive oil**

1 **teaspoon pure vanilla extract**

1 **cup fresh blueberries or other berries**

Position a rack in the center of the oven and preheat oven to 400°F. Lightly coat 24 nonstick miniature muffin cups with cooking oil spray.

In a medium bowl, combine the bran, flour, flaxseed, baking soda, cinnamon, and salt. Set aside. In another medium bowl or in a blender, combine the milk, honey, banana, egg, olive oil, and vanilla until smooth. Make a well in the center of the dry ingredients, and pour in one-third of the liquid mixture. Using a spoon, stir until smooth.

Add the remaining liquid mixture and stir just until combined. Add the blueberries and stir again, but do not overmix. Spoon 2 tablespoons of batter into each prepared muffin cup. Bake about 8 minutes, or until the tops spring back when pressed gently in the centers. Do not overbake. Cool in the pan on a wire rack for 10 minutes before removing from the cups. Serve warm or cool completely on the rack.

Make-Ahead Tip: To freeze these muffins for later use, wrap cooled muffins tightly in plastic wrap and place in freezer bags. Freeze for up to 3 months.

Blueberry Factoid: Color, not size, is an indicator of blueberry ripeness. Look for berries that are deep purple to blue-black.

Nutrient Analysis per muffin

76 calories; 3 g protein; 14 g carbohydrates; 2 g total fat; 0 g saturated fat; 1 g polyunsaturated fat; 1 g monounsaturated fat; 9 mg cholesterol; 2 g fiber; 85 mg sodium

SHANNON MULLEN'S EGG FOO YUNG

Yield: 2 servings

In the 1950s, this Chinese omelette was a popular dish in westernized Chinese restaurants. Made with various vegetables, it also contained meat or shrimp and was sometimes deep-fried. This lighter version is great for a special breakfast, brunch, or lunch.

½   cup finely shredded cabbage or fresh bean sprouts, rinsed and drained

¼   cup thinly sliced mushrooms

¼   cup finely sliced (or grated) carrots

2   tablespoons finely sliced green onions

2   tablespoons chopped red bell pepper

1   teaspoon chopped garlic

1   teaspoon chopped fresh ginger

6   large egg whites and 1 whole egg (or 1¼ cups egg substitute)

⅔   cup diced lean turkey, about 4 ounces (or chicken, lean pork, or cooked shrimp)

½   teaspoon black pepper

1   tablespoon chopped fresh cilantro or green onion Low-sodium soy sauce

Lightly coat a large nonstick sauté pan with cooking oil spray. Over medium-high heat, sauté the cabbage or sprouts, mushrooms, carrots, onions, bell pepper, garlic, and ginger for about 3 minutes or until almost tender but still bright. Transfer vegetables to a bowl to cool. Clean sauté pan to use again.

Beat the eggs well. Add the turkey, vegetables, and black pepper. Stir to combine.

Again, lightly coat the pan with cooking oil spray and place over medium-high heat. When the pan is hot, add the egg foo yung mixture. Cook for 1 minute, until it is set around the edges. Reduce heat to low, cover and simmer for 2 to 3 minutes or until eggs are set in middle.

Remove from heat, cover, and allow to rest for 2 minutes. Fold eggs in half and then cut in half again before transferring to two large plates. Garnish with fresh cilantro or green onion and serve hot with low-sodium soy sauce.

Ginger Factoid: Ginger contains an antioxidant called *gingerol,* which stimulates the gall bladder and enhances digestion.

Nutrient Analysis per serving
169 calories; 24 g protein; 9 g carbohydrates; 4 g total fat; 1 g saturated fat; 1 g polyunsaturated fat; 1 g monounsaturated fat; 129 mg cholesterol; 2 g fiber; 396 mg sodium

AARON SEMMEL'S OMELETTE OF CHAMPIONS

Yield: 1 serving

"While the omelette is cooking, I mix a smoothie in the blender and cook a little turkey bacon on the side."

4	**tablespoons chopped broccoli**
2	**tablespoons chopped yellow onion**
2	**tablespoons finely chopped carrot**
4	**large egg whites**
1	**whole large egg**
½	**teaspoon Mrs. Dash**
1	**ounce Light Laughing Cow cheese**
2	**tablespoons fat-free refried beans**

Lightly coat a medium nonstick sauté pan with cooking oil spray.

Heat the pan over medium-high heat and add the broccoli, onion, and carrot. Sauté for about 2 minutes or until just tender, but still bright. While the veggies are cooking, whip the eggs with a whisk or beater until they are foamy and light. Add the seasoning. Pour the eggs over the vegetables, cover, and cook for about 2 minutes or until the eggs are almost set.

Crumble the cheese over the omelette. Distribute the refried beans over the cheese. Fold the omelette in half and allow to cook 2 minutes longer over low heat.

When you are finished, head for the gym.

Broccoli Factoid: Broccoli contains a compound called *sulforaphanc,* which has shown promising anticancer effects. Current studies are now focusing on broccoli sprouts due to their particularly high antioxidant activity.

Nutrient Analysis per serving
247 calories; 28 g protein; 14 g carbohydrates; 8 g total fat; 3 g saturated fat; 1 g polyunsaturated fat; 2 g monounsaturated fat; 212 mg cholesterol; 3 g fiber; 783 mg sodium

DANA DESILVIO'S YOGURT PARFAIT

Yield: 1 serving

If you don't have fresh strawberries, other fresh berries work well. And if fresh berries are out of season, dried berries will work, but use only 2 tablespoons.

¼ **cup diced fresh strawberries**

2 **tablespoons low-fat granola**

1 **cup low-fat vanilla yogurt (8 ounces)**

Fresh mint sprig

Place the strawberries and granola in a small mixing bowl and stir to combine.

Spoon half of the mixture into a serving dish or parfait glass. Spoon the yogurt over the granola mixture. Sprinkle the remaining granola-strawberry mixture on top. Garnish with fresh mint.

Strawberry Factoid: The size of a strawberry does not determine its flavor. All strawberries large or small can be equally delicious if grown and harvested properly and if eaten at the height of ripeness.

Nutrient Analysis per serving
253 calories; 13 g protein; 44 g carbohydrates; 4 g total fat; 2 g saturated fat; 0 g polyunsaturated fat; 1 g monounsaturated fat; 11 mg cholesterol; 2 g fiber; 172 mg sodium

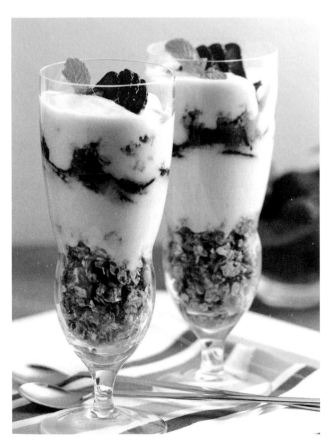

lunch

BARBECUE LENTILS

Yield: 1 quart; 8 (½-cup) servings

Quick and easy, this barbecue favorite is absolutely addictive. A great make-ahead dish for a potluck or a picnic, it's loaded with fiber.

1	tablespoon olive oil
1	cup chopped red onion
1	tablespoon minced garlic
2	teaspoons chili powder
1	teaspoon mustard powder
2	cups fat-free chicken or vegetable broth
¾	cup tomato sauce
3	tablespoons balsamic vinegar
1	tablespoon Dijon mustard
2	tablespoons agave nectar or honey
1½	cups dried (uncooked) brown lentils, rinsed
	Salt and freshly ground black pepper, to taste

Heat the oil in a 2-quart saucepan over medium heat. Add the onion and sauté until softened and translucent, about 3 minutes. Add the garlic, chili powder, and mustard powder and sauté until fragrant, about 1 minute; do not brown the garlic. Add the broth, tomato sauce, vinegar, mustard, agave nectar or honey, and lentils; stir well, and bring to a boil. Reduce heat to low, cover, and simmer until the lentils are tender, but intact, about 30 minutes.

Lentil cooking times vary. If necessary, add ¼ cup water and simmer for 5 minutes longer if lentils are not tender. Season with salt and pepper.

Lentil Factoid: Lentils are very high in folate. One cup of cooked lentils provides 90 percent of the daily recommended intake for adults.

Nutrient Analysis per serving
187 calories; 12 g protein; 31 g carbohydrates; 2 g total fat; 0 g saturated fat; less than 1 g polyunsaturated fat; 1 g monounsaturated fat; 0 mg cholesterol; 9 g fiber; 161 mg sodium

LISA ANDREONE'S WILD RICE AND TOASTED ALMONDS

Yield: 6 (1-cup) servings

Start this recipe on the stovetop and pop it in the oven while you finish cooking the rest of your meal.

1	teaspoon olive oil
1	cup wild rice, rinsed and drained
½	cup sliced mushrooms
½	cup chopped yellow onion
2	tablespoons chopped almonds (or almond meal)
1	tablespoon minced garlic
2	teaspoons chopped fresh thyme (or 1 teaspoon dried)
2	cups fat-free chicken or vegetable broth
½	cup water

Preheat the oven to 375°F. In a large nonstick sauté pan, heat the oil over medium heat. Add the rice, mushrooms, onion, almonds, garlic, and thyme. Cook about 5 minutes, stirring constantly, until the mixture is fragrant and the onion is just starting to soften. Do not allow the garlic or nuts to brown. Transfer mixture to a 2-quart baking dish. Meanwhile, bring the broth and water to a boil and pour over the rice mixture in the baking dish. Cover with foil and bake 1 hour. Serve hot.

Wild Rice Factoid: Wild rice is a great source of protein, B vitamins, iron, and fiber—and its nutty flavor is a delicious way to enjoy whole grains.

Nutrient Analysis per serving
156 calories; 7 g protein; 25 g carbohydrates; 4 g total fat; less than 1 g saturated fat; less than 1 g polyunsaturated fat; 2 g monounsaturated fat; 0 mg cholesterol; 3 g fiber; 162 mg sodium

DAVE FIORAVANTI'S GRILLED CHICKEN SALAD

Yield: 4 servings

Dave loves to make this easy and delicious recipe whenever he has last-minute guests. It's no wonder they keep dropping by at dinnertime!

8	**cups shredded romaine lettuce**
1	**yellow bell pepper, seeded and diced**
1	**cup diced cucumber**
½	**cup Salsa Vinaigrette (see page 157)**
4	**grilled boneless, skinless chicken breasts (cooked weight about 4 ounces each)**
½	**cup Creamy Hummus (see page 146)**
2	**tablespoons chopped fresh parsley or cilantro**

Place the romaine, pepper, and cucumber in a large mixing bowl. Add the salsa vinaigrette. Toss well.

Divide the salad evenly among four dinner plates. Place one grilled chicken breast on top of each salad. Top each chicken breast with 2 tablespoons of hummus. Garnish with parsley or cilantro. Serve immediately.

Tomato Factoid: If you're out of tomato sauce, you can convert a 3-ounce can of tomato paste into sauce by adding 1 cup of water.

Nutrient Analysis per serving
278 calories; 39 g protein; 11 g carbohydrates; 8 g total fat; 2 g saturated fat; 1 g polyunsaturated fat; 4 g monounsaturated fat; 86 mg cholesterol; 3 g fiber; 270 mg sodium

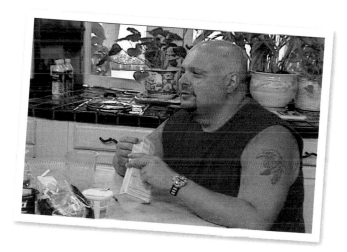

SETH WORD'S ROAST BEEF MELT

Yield: 1 sandwich

If your market doesn't have Ezekiel bread, look for a good multigrain bread with lots of fiber.

2	slices Ezekiel bread
2	slices fat-free American cheese
4	ounces lean deli thin-sliced roast beef
1	tablespoon brown mustard
3	thin slices yellow onion

Toast the Ezekiel bread on the grill with the cheese slices on top until the cheese melts. Put the roast beef on the toast. Top with the mustard and onion slices. Enjoy!

Onion Factoid: Eye tearing caused by cutting onions can be prevented by chilling them beforehand. The cold inactivates the offending compound (*propanethial-s-oxide*) and prevents it from becoming airborne.

Nutrient Analysis per sandwich
348 calories; 37 g protein; 37 g carbohydrates; 5 g total fat; 1 g saturated fat; 1 g polyunsaturated fat; 2 g monounsaturated fat; 55 mg cholesterol; 7 g fiber; 470 mg sodium

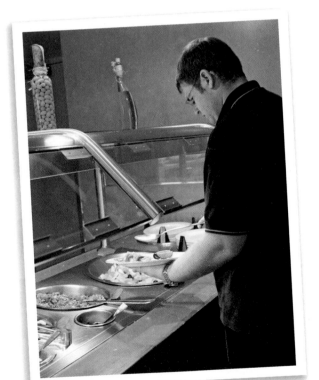

ICY GAZPACHO

Yield: 1½ quarts; 4 (1½-cup) servings

The southern region of Spain is the birthplace of this refreshing summer favorite. The sweetness of plump ripened tomatoes mingles with the fresh flavors of garden vegetables, cilantro, and a hint of balsamic vinegar. Toss 4 ounces of cooked shrimp in each serving, add a salad, and you have lunch.

1   **large red bell pepper**

2   **large tomatoes or 6 plum tomatoes (about 1 pound)**

1   **large cucumber, peeled, halved lengthwise, and seeded**

½   **medium yellow onion**

1   **cup tomato juice**

½   **cup chopped fresh cilantro, without stems**

¼   **cup balsamic vinegar**

2   **tablespoons fresh lime juice**

     Salt and freshly ground black pepper, to taste

Roast the bell pepper whole under the broiler or over a gas flame, turning occasionally, until the skin blisters and chars all over. Place in a bowl, cover with a lid, and let the steam loosen the skin, or place in a paper bag until it is just cool enough to handle. Carefully peel away the skin and remove the seeds. Cut the pepper into medium dice and set aside.

Cut half of the tomatoes, half of the cucumber, and half of the onion into 1-inch pieces and transfer to the bowl of a food processor or a blender jar. Add the roasted bell pepper and process to a puree. Transfer mixture to a medium mixing bowl. Add the tomato juice, cilantro, and vinegar. Seed the remaining tomato. Cut remaining tomato, cucumber, and onion into medium dice and add to the soup.

Refrigerate until chilled. Add the lime juice before serving and season with salt and black pepper. Serve well chilled. For a less chunky gazpacho, thin with additional tomato juice.

Tomato Factoid: Juicing tomatoes that haven't been cooked results in separation of the juice due to an enzyme that is activated when tomatoes are cut or crushed. Cooking the tomatoes first inactivates the enzyme, and the juiced tomatoes won't separate.

Nutrient Analysis per serving
63 calories; 2 g protein; 14 g carbohydrates; less than 1 g total fat; 0 g saturated fat; 0 g polyunsaturated fat; less than 1 g monounsaturated fat; 0 mg cholesterol; 3 g fiber; 15 mg sodium

SALAD ROMESCO

Yield: 6 servings

Romesco is a classic Spanish sauce of roasted peppers, tomato, almonds, garlic, and olive oil. It is usually served on bread or pasta. This recipe converts the classic sauce to a vinaigrette by staying true to the ingredients, but tweaking the proportions with more vinegar and less oil. Wonderful on crisp baby greens, the dressing is also delicious as a sauce or a dip for roasted or grilled vegetables.

FOR THE DRESSING:

1	medium red bell pepper
¼	cup almonds, toasted (see note)
3	cloves garlic, peeled
1	teaspoon grated lemon peel
¼	cup red wine vinegar or balsamic vinegar
⅓	cup extra-virgin olive oil
	Salt and freshly ground black pepper, to taste

FOR THE SALAD:

6	cups baby spinach, rinsed and dried
1½	cups cherry tomatoes (about 8 ounces), quartered
1	cup diced, seeded cucumber
¼	cup sliced, pitted kalamata olives
1	tablespoon finely chopped fresh oregano
1	tablespoon finely chopped fresh mint leaves
	Salt and freshly ground black pepper, to taste

Prepare the dressing: Roast the bell pepper whole under a broiler or over a gas flame, turning occasionally, until the skin blisters and chars all over. Place in a bowl, cover with a lid, and let the steam loosen the skin. When it is just cool enough to handle, remove from bowl and carefully peel away the skin and remove the seeds. Cut the pepper into medium dice and place in the bowl of a food processor or blender.

Add the almonds, garlic, lemon peel, and vinegar. Process until smooth. With the machine running, add the olive oil in a thin stream through the feed tube; the sauce will thicken. Season with the salt and black pepper. There will be about 1 cup of dressing.

Prepare the salad: Combine the spinach, tomatoes, cucumber, olives, oregano, and mint in a large mixing bowl. Pour 3 tablespoons of the dressing over the salad and toss well. Season with salt and pepper. Serve immediately. Reserve extra dressing for another use.

Note: To toast almonds, spread the nuts on an ungreased baking sheet. Bake in a preheated 350°F oven about 6 minutes, stirring occasionally, or until golden brown.

Nutrient Analysis per serving
62 calories; 2 g protein; 5 g carbohydrates; 5 g total fat; less than 1 g saturated fat; less than 1 g polyunsaturated fat; 3 g monounsaturated fat; 0 mg cholesterol; 2 g fiber; 70 mg sodium

Bell Pepper Factoid: Green bell peppers are the most common type of bell pepper and are usually the least expensive. Red and yellow peppers stay on the vine longer, yielding more flavor and a higher price. No matter which color you favor, they're all rich sources of vitamin C.

TOMATO LENTIL SOUP

Yield: 1¼ quarts; 6 (¾-cup) servings

A traditional Indian soup, this can be made ahead and will keep well for 2 days refrigerated. It can also be frozen for up to 1 month.

½	**cup dried brown lentils**
4	**cups fat-free chicken or vegetable broth**
1	**tablespoon olive oil**
1½	**teaspoons black or yellow mustard seeds**
1	**pound plum tomatoes, peeled, seeded, and chopped**
3	**tablespoons peeled, finely chopped fresh ginger**
1	**clove garlic, minced**
1	**teaspoon ground coriander**
1	**teaspoon ground cumin**
1	**teaspoon ground turmeric**
	Pinch cinnamon
¼	**cup chopped fresh cilantro, without stems**
	Salt, to taste

Wash the lentils and drain well in a sieve. Add the lentils and 1½ cups of the broth to a 2-quart saucepan. Bring to a boil, reduce heat, and simmer lentils over low heat until they are tender, but still retain their shape, about 20 minutes.

Meanwhile, heat the oil in a heavy 4-quart saucepan over medium-high heat until hot but not smoking. Add the mustard seeds and cook, stirring, until the seeds just begin to pop. Carefully add the tomatoes, ginger, garlic, coriander, cumin, turmeric, and cinnamon. Simmer until the tomatoes are softened and the spices are fragrant, about 4 minutes. Add 1½ cups of the broth; bring to a boil. Reduce heat and simmer, stirring occasionally, for about 4 minutes.

Carefully transfer the tomato-ginger mixture to the bowl of a food processor or a blender jar. Process or blend until smooth. Return to the saucepan and add the cooked lentils and the remaining 1 cup of broth, stirring to incorporate. Bring the soup to a boil, stirring occasionally. Stir in the cilantro. Season to taste with salt.

Tomato Factoid: The official beverage of the state of Ohio is tomato juice.

Nutrient Analysis per serving
119 calories; 10 g protein; 14 g carbohydrates; 3 g total fat; 0 g saturated fat; 0 g polyunsaturated fat; 2 g monounsaturated fat; 0 mg cholesterol; 6 g fiber; 267 mg sodium

RYAN BENSON'S PORTOBELLO "PIZZAS"

Yield: 4 small pizzas

Most prefer to eat this "pizza" with a knife and fork!

4   **whole portobello mushroom caps (about 5 inches each), stems removed**

½   **cup low-fat marinara sauce**

½   **cup lean turkey Italian sausage, cooked, drained, and crumbled**

4   **tablespoons shredded fat-free or low-fat mozzarella cheese**

2   **teaspoons freshly grated Parmesan cheese**

1   **tablespoon chopped fresh basil**

Preheat the oven to 350°F. Wipe the mushrooms clean of any dirt. Place them on a baking sheet, gill side up. Spoon the sauce over each cap, then sprinkle on the sausage and the cheeses. Place in the oven and bake for 6 to 8 minutes, or until the cheese is melted. Garnish with fresh basil. Serve immediately.

Mushroom Factoid: One portobello mushroom has as much potassium as a banana.

Nutrient Analysis per pizza
97 calories; 10 g protein; 7 g carbohydrates; 3 g total fat; 1 g saturated fat; less than 1 g polyunsaturated fat; less than 1 g monounsaturated fat; 22 mg cholesterol; 2 g fiber; 305 mg sodium

dinner

CURRIED VEGETABLE STEW
Yield: 2 quarts; 8 (1-cup) servings

This robust stew is hearty enough for a main course. You can add extra broth to make a thinner soup. It's loaded with both protein and fiber.

1	tablespoon extra-virgin olive oil
1	medium red onion, finely chopped
1	medium green bell pepper, deseeded and finely chopped
½	cup chopped carrot
½	cup chopped celery
3	cloves garlic, minced
2	tablespoons peeled, minced fresh ginger
1	tablespoon curry powder
2	large tomatoes, peeled, seeded, and chopped, or 1 cup tomato sauce
1	bay leaf
4	cups fat-free chicken or vegetable broth
1½	cups cooked pinto beans or black beans
3	tablespoons creamy or crunchy natural peanut butter (or almond butter)
¼	cup chopped fresh cilantro
½	pound baby spinach leaves or other fresh greens, torn into bite-size pieces
	Salt and freshly ground black pepper, to taste

Heat the oil in a 4-quart saucepan or Dutch oven over medium heat. Add the onion, bell pepper, carrot, and celery and sauté until soft and translucent, about 5 minutes.

Add the garlic, ginger, and curry powder and sauté until fragrant; do not brown the garlic. Add the tomatoes or tomato sauce and bay leaf and cook, uncovered, until the tomatoes are slightly reduced, about 3 minutes.

Add the broth and bring the mixture to a boil. Reduce the heat to low. Stir in the beans and peanut butter until combined. Cook until heated through, about 2 minutes. Stir in the cilantro and spinach. Season with salt and black pepper. Serve immediately.

Peanut Factoid: Regular peanut butter contains a small amount of partially hydrogenated oil and trans fatty acids. This keeps the oil from separating out of the peanut butter, but like harmful cholesterol, it's not something we want lingering in our bloodstream. Natural peanut butters do not contain partially hydrogenated oils. The peanut oil rises to the top, but a quick stir will restore the peanut butter's creaminess.

Nutrient Analysis per serving
128 calories; 9 g protein; 16 g carbohydrates; 4 g total fat; 1 g saturated fat; 1 g polyunsaturated fat; 2 g monounsaturated fat; 0 mg cholesterol; 5 g fiber; 240 mg sodium

DOC'S CHILI
Yield: 10 servings

A simmering pot of Doc's Chili was found on the ranch stove every week during season two. The invention of Dr. Jeff Levine, this crowd-pleasing favorite is short on preparation time and long on flavor.

2	**20-ounce packages extra lean ground turkey breast**
2	**26-ounce jars Ragu Carb Options Garden Style Sauce**
1	**15.5-ounce can black beans, drained**
1	**15.5-ounce can red or pink beans, drained**
1	**15.5-ounce can pinto beans, drained**
1	**cup chopped onion**
1	**cup chopped green pepper**
1	**cup chopped red pepper**
1	**cup sliced mushrooms**
3	**tablespoons minced garlic**
3	**tablespoons black pepper**
3	**tablespoons chili powder**
3	**tablespoons fajita seasoning**

Brown the ground turkey in a nonstick 6–8 quart pot, breaking it into small pieces as it cooks. Drain any excess water. Add the sauce, black beans, red or pink beans, and pinto beans. Stir in the garlic, pepper, chili powder, fajita seasoning, onion, peppers, and mushrooms. Simmer, stirring occasionally, until the vegetables are cooked to desired tenderness.

Nutrient Analysis per serving
380 calories; 27 g protein; 12 g carbohydrates; 19 g total fat; 3.5 g saturated fat; 11 g fiber; 950 mg sodium

GARY DECKMAN'S FISH TACOS

Yield: About 8 stuffed tacos

"Here is my favorite dish right now . . . oh boy, is this good!"

FOR THE FISH:

1	pound orange roughy (or other boneless, skinless fish fillet such as red snapper)
3	tablespoons fresh lime juice
½	teaspoon paprika
½	teaspoon salt
½	teaspoon freshly ground black pepper
½	teaspoon chili powder (optional)

FOR THE TACOS:

8	whole-grain high-fiber tortillas (or stone-ground corn tortillas)
½	avocado, diced and lightly mashed
⅓	cup shredded low-fat Mexican cheeses (or pepper Jack)
½	cup tomato salsa
4	tablespoons chopped fresh cilantro
1½	cups finely shredded cabbage
	Hot sauce (optional)

Place the fish in a shallow baking dish. Sprinkle with the lime juice, paprika, salt, pepper, and chili powder (if using). Cover, refrigerate, and allow to marinate for about 30 minutes.

Preheat the grill to medium-high heat (or preheat oven to 375°F).

Lightly coat a 24 x 12-inch piece of aluminum foil with cooking oil spray. Place the fish in a single layer, in the center of the foil. Close the foil over to seal in the fish, folding the ends upward.

Place the foil packet on the preheated grill (or in preheated oven). Cook for about 7 to 10 minutes, or until the fish is opaque. Remove from the grill (or oven).

To assemble tacos: Wrap the tortillas in foil and place on the grill (or in oven) to warm for 2 minutes. Spread about ⅛ of the mashed avocado on each tortilla. Top with the fish. Sprinkle with the cheese, salsa, cilantro, and cabbage. Repeat for remaining tacos.

Serve with glasses of ice water garnished with a slice of orange and a sprig of fresh mint.

Fish Factoid: Orange roughy has a mild flavor and firm white flesh. It was first discovered off the coast of New Zealand but is now widely available.

Nutrient Analysis per 2 taco servings, using whole-grain high-fiber tortillas
300 calories; 37 g protein; 29 g carbohydrates; 11 g total fat; 3 g saturated fat; 2 g polyunsaturated fat; 6 g monounsaturated fat; 49 mg cholesterol; 9 g fiber; 611 mg sodium

MARK YESITIS'S GRILLED ITALIAN FLANK STEAK WITH ROMA TOMATOES

Yield: 4 servings

This is the epitome of a quick and easy dinner. Mix the marinade before work and when you come home, light the grill, toss a salad, and set the table—presto!

¼   cup balsamic vinegar

¼   cup water or low-sodium beef or chicken broth

1   tablespoon chopped garlic

1   tablespoon chopped fresh basil
     (or 1 teaspoon dried basil)

1   tablespoon chopped fresh thyme
     (or 1 teaspoon dried thyme)

1   teaspoon ground mustard seed

½   teaspoon freshly ground black pepper

1¼   pounds flank steak, trimmed of all visible fat

8   Roma tomatoes, halved crosswise

Combine the vinegar, water or broth, garlic, basil, thyme, mustard seed, and black pepper in a large zip-top plastic bag. Add the steak and seal the bag. Marinate refrigerated for at least 2 hours (but no longer than 12), turning the steak occasionally.

Prepare a fire in a charcoal grill or preheat a gas grill or broiler. Lightly coat the grill rack with cooking oil spray. Position the cooking rack 4 to 6 inches from the heat source.

Remove the steak from the marinade; drain and blot to remove excess marinade.

Place the steak and tomatoes on the grill rack or broiler pan. Grill or broil until browned, 4 or 5 minutes on each side for the steak and about 3 minutes on each side for the tomatoes. Watch the steak carefully as the balsamic vinegar can cause it to burn if not properly blotted. Check the steak for doneness by cutting into the meat. Let stand for 5 minutes on a cutting board. Cut the meat across the grain into very thin slices.

Roma Tomato Factoid: It takes 17 pounds of fresh tomatoes to make 1 pound of sun-dried tomatoes.

Nutrient Analysis per serving
241 calories; 25 g protein; 8 g carbohydrates; 11 g total fat; 5 g saturated fat; less than 1 g polyunsaturated fat; 5 g monounsaturated fat; 60 mg cholesterol; 2 g fiber; 72 mg sodium

PETE THOMAS'S SLIVERED PORK STIR-FRY WITH GARLIC, BROCCOLI, AND SESAME
Yield: 4 servings

Once you get the hang of it, it's easy to whip up stir-fries using any combination of your favorite veggies. Substitute lean beef or chicken for the pork, or switch seasonings—the combinations are endless.

3	**cups broccoli, chopped in 1-inch pieces**
¾	**cup chicken broth**
½	**cup chopped green onions**
2	**tablespoons chopped garlic**
2	**tablespoons peeled, chopped ginger**
2	**teaspoons olive oil**
1	**cup chopped yellow onion**
1	**red bell pepper, halved, seeded, and diced**
1	**pound boneless pork tenderloin, cut in thin strips ½ inch wide and 2 inches long (see note)**
1	**tablespoon low-sodium soy sauce**
1	**tablespoon toasted sesame seeds**

Steam the broccoli until bright green but still firm, about 2 minutes. Drain; rinse with cold water to stop the cooking; drain again. (If using frozen broccoli cuts, thaw the broccoli but omit this cooking step.)

Combine ¼ cup of the broth, the green onions, garlic, and ginger in a food processor or blender and pulse until the mixture is minced. Set aside.

Heat 1 teaspoon of the oil in a large nonstick sauté pan over medium-high heat. Add the onion and pepper; sauté 5 minutes or until the vegetables are just tender. Transfer to a bowl and cover with a towel to retain heat.

Add the remaining 1 teaspoon of oil to the pan over medium-high heat. Add the green onion mixture and sauté for about 1 minute, stirring constantly. Add the pork strips and soy sauce to the skillet and sauté for 4 minutes, or until pork is nearly cooked. Add the remaining ½ cup of broth and bring to a boil. Add the broccoli to skillet and stir until broccoli is cooked through, about 3 minutes. Add onion and bell pepper back to pan. Divide among four dinner plates and garnish with sesame seeds. Serve immediately.

Note: It's easier to slice pork thinly if you place it in the freezer for about 30 minutes first.

Nutrient Analysis per serving
259 calories; 29 g protein; 12 g carbohydrates; 10 g total fat; 3 g saturated fat; 2 g polyunsaturated fat; 5 g monounsaturated fat; 78 mg cholesterol; 4 g fiber; 280 mg sodium

Green Onion Factoid: Also known as scallions, green onions have a milder flavor than onions, can be eaten raw or cooked, and can be used as a garnish or an ingredient.

SUZY PRESTON'S RANCH-STYLE "SPAGHETTI" MARINARA

Yield: 4 servings

This flavorful squash can always be found in the kitchen at the ranch as a creative replacement for white pasta. Add turkey meatballs and a salad and you have a meal.

1	**medium spaghetti squash (about 1½ pounds)**
2	**cups low-fat marinara sauce**
2	**tablespoons chopped fresh basil or parsley**
2	**tablespoons grated Romano or Parmesan cheese**

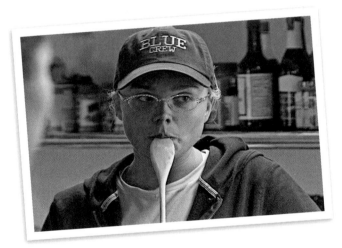

Preheat the oven to 375°F. Lightly coat a baking sheet with cooking oil spray.

Wash the outside of the squash and cut it in half lengthwise. Remove the seeds. Pierce the outside of each half a few times with a fork. Place the squash cut side down on the baking sheet and bake until very tender when tested with a fork, about 45 minutes. Cool slightly.

Meanwhile, heat the marinara sauce and keep it warm.

Using the tines of a fork, rake the spaghetti-like threads of the squash into a mixing bowl. Discard the skin. There will be about 3 cups of spaghetti squash. Pour the hot marinara sauce over the squash and toss gently.

Divide the "spaghetti" among four serving plates and garnish with basil or parsley and cheese.

Squash Factoid: Remember to pierce the squash with a fork before baking or it may explode in the oven.

Nutrient Analysis per serving
114 calories; 4 g protein; 18 g carbohydrates; 4 g total fat; 1 g saturated fat; 1 g polyunsaturated fat; 1 g monounsaturated fat; 2 mg cholesterol; 4 g fiber; 574 mg sodium

SUZANNE MENDONCA'S GRILLED SALMON BURGERS

Yield: 4 servings

These burgers are a delicious way to enjoy fish rich in omega-3s. If you don't have a grill, they can also be cooked in a large, nonstick sauté pan over medium-high heat.

1	**pound skinless salmon fillet, cut into 1-inch dice**
1	**tablespoon Dijon mustard**
1	**tablespoon grated lime peel**
1	**tablespoon peeled, minced fresh ginger**
1	**tablespoon chopped fresh cilantro**
1	**teaspoon low-sodium soy sauce**
½	**teaspoon ground coriander**
	Salt and freshly ground black pepper, to taste
	Fresh lime wedges and cilantro sprigs

Lightly coat a grill rack with cooking oil spray. Preheat the grill to medium hot.

In the bowl of a food processor, pulse the salmon just enough to grind it coarsely. Transfer the salmon to a large bowl and mix in the mustard, lime peel, ginger, cilantro, soy sauce, and coriander. Form the salmon mixture into four patties and season with salt and pepper.

Grill the burgers, turning once, until done, 4 minutes per side for medium doneness.

Garnish with fresh lime wedges and cilantro sprigs and serve.

Salmon Factoid: High amounts of omega-3s are found in fish such as salmon, tuna, and mackerel because they feed on plankton, an organism that produces those fatty acids.

Nutrient Analysis per serving
194 calories; 26 g protein; 2 g carbohydrates; 8 g total fat; 1 g saturated fat; 3 g polyunsaturated fat; 3 g monounsaturated fat; 72 mg cholesterol; less than 1 g fiber; 243 mg sodium

snacks

ANDREA BAPTISTE'S BAKED CORN CHIPS
Yield: 12 eight-chip servings

Plain or seasoned, corn chips are great to have on hand when you have the urge to crunch. Great with salsa or Edamame Guacamole (see opposite page), they're best eaten when just baked, but they can also be stored in an airtight plastic bag.

12	**6-inch stone-ground corn tortillas (about 12 ounces)**
¼	**teaspoon ground cumin (optional)**
¼	**teaspoon chili powder (optional)**
¼	**teaspoon salt (optional)**

Preheat the oven to 350°F.

Divide the tortillas into two stacks. Cut each stack into eight chip-size wedges. Arrange the chips in a single layer on two baking sheets. Lightly coat chips with olive oil cooking spray. Sprinkle with cumin, chili powder, and salt, if using. Gently toss the chips and rearrange to cover the baking sheets evenly.

Bake for 10 minutes. Rotate the baking sheets and bake for 10 minutes longer or until the chips are crisp, but not brown. (Keep in mind that fresh tortillas have more moisture and will take a few minutes longer to bake than not-so-fresh tortillas.) Cool. Serve.

Cooking Oil Spray Factoid: Don't use aerosolized cans. It's tastier and less expensive to make your own cooking oil spray (and it's easy, too!). Spray bottles are available in health food stores and can be filled with your own fresh oils as needed. For regular baking and sautéing, fill the spray bottle with a mild-flavored oil. Vegetable oils can be stored in a cool, dark place for up to 4 months.

Nutrient Analysis per serving
64 calories; 1 g protein; 12 g carbohydrates; 1 g total fat; 0 g saturated fat; 0 g polyunsaturated fat; 1 g monounsaturated fat; 0 mg cholesterol; 2 g fiber; 42 mg sodium

EDAMAME GUACAMOLE

Yield: 2 cups; 16 (2-tablespoon) servings

This delicious imposter has 30 percent fewer calories and fat than traditional guacamole, plus more protein, greater nutrient diversity, and lots of isoflavones.

1	**cup shelled edamame (about 12 ounces unshelled)**
½	**cup unflavored soymilk**
2	**tablespoons chopped fresh cilantro, without stems**
2	**cloves garlic, minced**
1	**teaspoon chopped chipotle chile pepper (optional)**
1	**large ripe avocado**
2	**teaspoons fresh lime juice**
	Salt and freshly ground black pepper, to taste
1	**tablespoon chopped fresh cilantro, without stems**

Cook the edamame in salted boiling water for 5 minutes. Drain and cool to room temperature.

Combine the edamame, soymilk, cilantro, garlic, and chile pepper, if using, in the bowl of a food processor. Process until mixture is very smooth, about 3 minutes. Set aside.

Peel and seed the avocado and place in a medium mixing bowl. Add the lime juice and mash with a fork, leaving small chunks. Add the edamame mixture and stir just to combine. Season with salt and black pepper. Garnish with cilantro.

Edamame Factoid: In addition to being a great snack, 1 cup of cooked edamame has 7 grams of fiber and a whopping 22 grams of protein.

Nutrient Analysis per serving
45 calories; 3 g protein; 3 g carbohydrates; 3 g total fat; less than 1 g saturated fat; 1 g polyunsaturated fat; 0 g monounsaturated fat; 0 mg cholesterol; 2 g fiber; 4 mg sodium

CREAMY HUMMUS

Yield: About 2 cups; 16 (2-tablespoon) servings

This creamy Middle Eastern spread takes minutes to prepare and will keep for several days, refrigerated. Serve as a snack with raw veggies, use as an omelette filling, or try it with Dave Fioravanti's Grilled Chicken Salad (see page 131).

3	cups cooked chickpeas or 2 (15-ounce) cans, drained and rinsed
½	cup warm water
3	tablespoons fresh lime juice
1	tablespoon tahini
1½	teaspoons ground cumin
1	tablespoon minced garlic
1	teaspoon salt
2	tablespoons chopped fresh cilantro

Place the chickpeas, water, lime juice, tahini, cumin, garlic, and salt in the bowl of a food processor. Process until very smooth, about 4 minutes. Add an extra tablespoon or two of water if necessary. Transfer to a bowl. Stir in fresh cilantro.

Chickpea Factoid: Also called garbanzo beans are firm, round, beige beans used extensively in Middle Eastern, Indian, and Mediterranean cuisine. One ½-cup serving of chickpeas has 7 grams of protein, 6 grams of fiber, and 60 milligrams of calcium.

Nutrient Analysis per serving
54 calories; 3 g protein; 8 g carbohydrates; 1 g total fat; less than 1 g saturated fat; less than 1 g polyunsaturated fat; 1 g monounsaturated fat; 0 mg cholesterol; 2 g fiber; 112 mg sodium

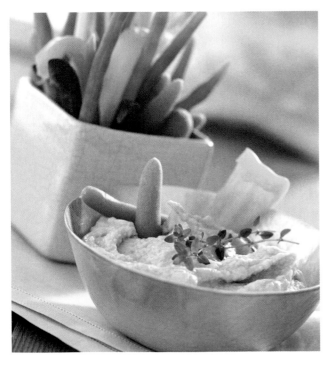

LIZZETH DAVALOS'S PITA PIZZA
Yield: 1 pizza

The joy of this recipe is that it's just as easy to make one for yourself as it is to make several for a last-minute get-together. Be sure to use whole wheat pitas—they're great to have on hand and store well in the freezer.

2	**tablespoons low-fat pizza sauce**
1	**whole wheat pita bread (approx. 6 inches)**
1	**ounce thinly sliced turkey**
1	**tablespoon chopped yellow onion**
1	**tablespoon chopped bell pepper**
1	**tablespoon finely diced pineapple**
2	**tablespoons shredded fat-free mozzarella cheese**

Preheat the oven to 425°F.

Spread the pizza sauce over the pita bread. Top with the turkey, onion, pepper, and pineapple. Sprinkle with the shredded cheese.

Place the pita on a baking sheet and bake for about 8 minutes, or until the pita bread has reached the desired crispness and the cheese is melted.

Whole Wheat Factoid: In addition to more fiber and antioxidants, whole wheat breads naturally have more vitamin E, B vitamins, and micronutrients than their refined white counterparts.

Nutrient Analysis per pizza
204 calories; 15 g protein; 33 g carbohydrates; 3 g total fat; less than 1 g saturated fat; less than 1 g polyunsaturated fat; less than 1 g monounsaturated fat; 14 mg cholesterol; 6 g fiber; 555 mg sodium

THE KELLY MAC SNACK

Yield: 1 serving

"I don't really make any exciting food items that are original. I do make this snack thing that I try to eat instead of an energy bar. It's called the Kelly Mac Snack. It's the same calories as a bar, except more natural."

22   **dry-roasted unsalted almonds**

1   **tablespoon dark chocolate chips**

2   **tablespoons raisins**

Put the almonds, chocolate chips, and raisins in a little snack bag and pop it in your bag for the day. Try not to get stuck eating energy bars on the go.

Almond Factoid: A compound called flavonoids in almond skins may be responsible for the nuts' positive effect on cholesterol levels.

Nutrient Analysis per serving
210 calories; 5 g protein; 25 g carbohydrates; 12 g total fat; 2 g saturated fat; 2 g polyunsaturated fat; 7 g monounsaturated fat; 0 mg cholesterol; 3 g fiber; 8 mg sodium

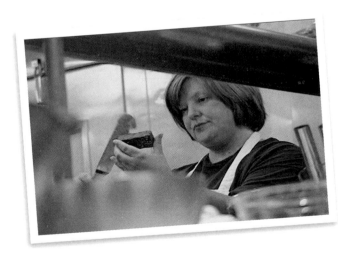

MATT KAMONT'S ROAST ASPARAGUS WITH SMOKED SALMON

Yield: 4 four-spear servings

This easy recipe is elegant enough to serve as an hors d'oeuvre, yet simple enough for a snack. Thicker asparagus spears are easier to handle for wrapping.

1   **pound asparagus, tough ends snapped (about 16 medium spears)**

2   **teaspoons extra-virgin olive oil**
     Sea salt and freshly ground black pepper, to taste

4   **thin slices smoked salmon (about 4 ounces), each cut in 4 lengthwise strips**

Preheat the oven to 425°F. Place the asparagus spears on a baking sheet so they are not touching. Drizzle the spears with the oil and sprinkle with salt and pepper. Roast for 5 to 10 minutes, turning once, until tender crisp. Do not overcook or they will be too soft and difficult to handle. When the spears are cool enough to handle, wrap each spear with a very thin slice of smoked salmon. Serve immediately or chill to serve later.

This recipe also works well with grilled asparagus spears.

Salmon Factoid: The healthy omega-3 fats found in salmon are thought to improve heart health and reduce inflammation.

Nutrient Analysis per serving
85 calories; 8 g protein; 5 g carbohydrates; 3 g total fat; 1 g saturated fat; 1 g polyunsaturated fat; 1 g monounsaturated fat; 7 mg cholesterol; 2 g fiber; 222 mg sodium

ANDREA OVERSTREET'S TURKEY WRAP

Yield: 2 one-wrap servings

"Butter lettuce instead of a bun is my favorite way to save calories!"

6	ounces 99 percent fat-free ground turkey breast
	Salt and freshly ground black pepper, to taste
2	leaves butter lettuce
8	thin slices cucumber
2	tablespoons fresh alfalfa sprouts
2	tablespoons fresh bean sprouts
2	tablespoons low-fat miso Caesar dressing

Form the turkey into a patty, about 4½ inches in diameter. Season the patty with the salt and pepper and grill until cooked, about 3 or 4 minutes on each side.

Cut the patty in half and place each half in the center of one of the butter lettuce leaves. Top burgers with the cucumber and alfalfa and bean sprouts. Drizzle with the dressing, and wrap the lettuce around the burger and vegetables.

Butter Lettuce Factoid: Also called Bibb lettuce or Boston lettuce, butter lettuce has a mild, delicate flavor.

Nutrient Analysis per wrap
145 calories; 18 g protein; 4 g carbohydrates; 7 g total fat; 2 g saturated fat; 2 g polyunsaturated fat; 2 g monounsaturated fat; 61 mg cholesterol; 1 g fiber; 224 mg sodium

MATT HOOVER'S CHIPOTLE CHICKEN

Yield: 1 serving

Matt's a no-nonsense kind of cook. This is one of his favorite snacks after a tough workout.

1	**8-ounce boneless, skinless chicken breast**
	Chipotle Tabasco Sauce, to taste
½	**teaspoon garlic salt**

Lightly coat a grill rack with cooking oil spray. Preheat the grill to medium hot.

Grill the chicken until done, about 4 minutes per side. Season with the chipotle sauce and garlic salt. Enjoy!

Chipotle Factoid: Chipotle is a smoked jalapeño chile. It imparts a rich, smoky taste when used as a flavoring. It's very hot, so a little dab'll do ya.

Nutrient Analysis per serving
250 calories; 52 g protein; 0 g carbohydrates; 3 g total fat; 1 g saturated fat; 1 g polyunsaturated fat; 1 g monounsaturated fat; 132 mg cholesterol; 0 g fiber; 602 mg sodium

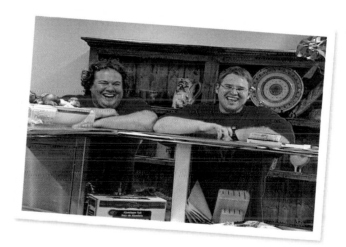

RYAN KELLY'S PITA TRIANGLES

Yield: 12 eight-triangle servings

Whole wheat pita bread is great to keep on hand. These are easy to throw together for last-minute entertaining. Add a bowl of Creamy Hummus (see page 146) and let the party begin!

6	**6-inch whole wheat pita breads**
¾	**teaspoon garlic powder, onion powder, or a seasoning such as Mrs. Dash**

Preheat the oven to 375°F.

With a sharp knife, cut each pita bread in half, then each half into 4 triangles. Carefully separate each triangle into 2 pieces. There should be 16 small triangles per pita bread.

Arrange the triangles in a single layer on two baking sheets. Lightly coat the triangles with olive oil cooking spray. Sprinkle with the seasoning of your choice. Gently toss and rearrange to cover the baking sheets.

Bake for 5 minutes. Remove from oven, and using a metal spatula, gently turn the pitas over. Continue to bake until crisp and golden brown, about 8 minutes longer. Chips will get crispy as they cool. Store in airtight containers or self-sealing plastic bags.

Pita Bread Factoid: Pita bread is made from a wheat dough that is leavened with yeast. Thin rounds of flat dough are baked at a high temperature, causing the dough to rise quickly and dramatically during baking. When it cools, steam leaves an air pocket that is perfect for stuffing sandwiches.

Nutrient Analysis per serving
92 calories; 3 g protein; 18 g carbohydrates; 2 g total fat; 0 g saturated fat; less than 1 g polyunsaturated fat; less than 1 g monounsaturated fat; 0 mg cholesterol; 2 g fiber; 170 mg sodium

KELLY MINNER'S CREAM CHEESE ROLL-UPS

Yield: 2 servings

"This is a great snack to make when you need something simple but satisfying. You can also make them ahead so they're good to go when you need a nibble in a hurry. I prefer the low-fat Lebanon bologna."

2   **slices roast turkey or turkey bologna (2 ounces)**

2   **tablespoons fat-free cream cheese with chives (or garden vegetable flavor)**

Place the meat slices on a flat surface. Spread thinly with the cream cheese. Roll tightly. Cover and refrigerate until use.

Turkey Factoid: One ounce of lean turkey has the same amount of protein as two large egg whites (about 7 grams).

Nutrient Analysis per serving
73 calories; 5 g protein; 2 g carbohydrates; 5 g total fat; 1 g saturated fat; 1 g polyunsaturated fat; 2 g monounsaturated fat; 22 mg cholesterol; less than 1 g fiber; 434 mg sodium

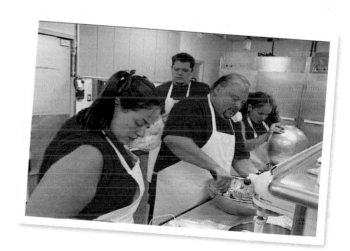

other

JEN KERSEY'S PEANUTTY SPREAD

Yield: 1½ cups; 12 (2-tablespoon) servings

Blending creamy peanut butter with silky tofu cuts the calories and fat by nearly two-thirds. It's the perfect high-protein snack whether spread on a whole grain cracker or used as a dip for apple slices or raw veggies. And one dollop makes a wickedly good topping for your favorite fat-free chocolate pudding . . .

1	**cup silky tofu, drained (about 9 ounces)**
⅓	**cup peanut butter**
4	**teaspoons honey**
2	**teaspoons lime juice**

Place the tofu, peanut butter, honey, and lime juice in a blender or a food processor. Blend or process until smooth. Add a few teaspoons of water if necessary. Store in the refrigerator.

Tofu Factoid: Tofu is made from soymilk, similar to the way cheese is made from dairy milk. It has a neutral taste and easily absorbs the flavors of other ingredients it is mixed with.

Nutrient Analysis per serving

80 calories; 5 g protein; 4 g carbohydrates; 5 g total fat; 1 g saturated fat; 1 g polyunsaturated fat; 3 g monounsaturated fat; 0 mg cholesterol; 1 g fiber; 36 mg sodium

KATHRYN MURPHY'S EASY RASPBERRY SORBET

Yield: 4 servings

"I can't cook" is no excuse to not make this simple treat. The sky's the limit for flavor possibilities because you can use different berries or fruits, such as peaches or mango.

2	**cups frozen raspberries (or other frozen fruit)**
3	**tablespoons apple juice or orange juice**
½	**teaspoon cinnamon or vanilla extract (optional)**
	Fresh mint leaves

Place the fruit, juice, and cinnamon or vanilla, if using, in a blender or a food processor. Blend or process until smooth, scraping down the sides of the container as necessary. Add extra juice if needed. Best if served immediately, although it can be frozen. Garnish with fresh mint.

Raspberry Factoid: Raspberries contain a compound called ellagic acid, which has been found to promote wound healing and fight heart disease.

Nutrient Analysis per serving
37 calories; 1 g protein; 9 g carbohydrates; 0 g total fat; 0 g saturated fat; 0 g polyunsaturated fat; 0 g monounsaturated fat; 0 mg cholesterol; 4 g fiber; 1 mg sodium

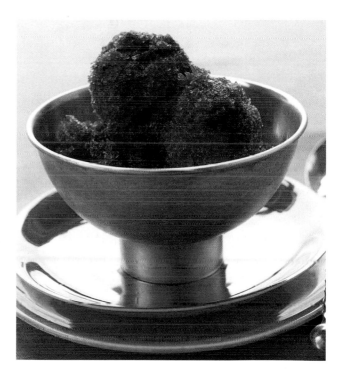

TANGY TAHINI MUSTARD SAUCE

Yield: 2 cups; 32 (1-tablespoon) servings

This tangy sauce is an addictive condiment. Try it with Suzanne Mendonca's Grilled Salmon Burgers (see page 143) or on your own favorite sandwich. It will keep for several weeks in the refrigerator—if it lasts that long.

⅔ **cup Dijon mustard**

½ **cup tahini**

½ **cup soft silken tofu**

⅓ **cup fresh lemon juice**

Combine the mustard, tahini, tofu, and lemon juice in a blender and blend until smooth. For a thinner sauce, add 1 or 2 tablespoons of water. Pour into an airtight container and refrigerate.

Tahini Factoid: Sesame seeds are commonly ground into pastes. Those with thicker textures are referred to as sesame butter; thinner pastes are called tahini.

Nutrient Analysis per serving
32 calories; 1 g protein; 2 g carbohydrates; 3 g total fat; 0 g saturated fat; 1 g polyunsaturated fat; 1 g monounsaturated fat; 0 mg cholesterol; 0 g fiber; 128 mg sodium

MO WALKER'S SALSA VINAIGRETTE

Yield: 1 cup; 16 (1-tablespoon) servings

This vinaigrette is delicious on a piece of fish or chicken or tossed with beans, whole grains, or a green salad. Try different vinegars or add herbs for new flavors.

1	**cup roasted tomato salsa (or your favorite salsa)**
¼	**cup cider vinegar**
3	**tablespoons extra-virgin olive oil**
½	**teaspoon freshly ground black pepper**

Combine the salsa, vinegar, oil, and pepper in a blender or food processor and blend or process until smooth. There will be about 1 cup of vinaigrette.

Olive Oil Factoid: Buying a large bottle with a proportionately better price tag is not the best option if you use oil infrequently. When in doubt of your oil's freshness, throw it out and open a fresh bottle. Even 1 tablespoon of rancid oil can ruin the flavor of an entire recipe.

Nutrient Analysis per serving
28 calories; less than 1 g protein; 1 g carbohydrates; 3 g total fat; less than 1 g saturated fat; less than 1 g polyunsaturated fat; 2 g monounsaturated fat; 0 mg cholesterol; 0 g fiber; 70 mg sodium

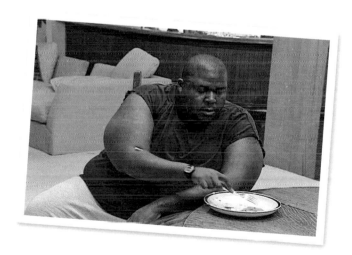

MINT TEA

Yield: 4 cups; 4 (1-cup) servings

Hot mint tea is served throughout the day in Morocco. It's also delicious iced.

2	**tablespoons loose-leaf green tea or 3 green-tea bags**
¾	**cup lightly packed fresh mint leaves**
1	**teaspoon grated lemon peel**
4	**cups boiling water**

Place the tea, mint leaves, and lemon peel in a pot or small saucepan and add the boiling water. Cover and allow to steep for 8 minutes. Using a strainer, pour the tea into small cups or heat-proof glasses.

Tea Factoid: Tea bags contain broken tea leaves that are smaller and have a greater surface area than loose tea. They produce an infusion with more caffeine than loose tea does.

Nutrient Analysis per serving
1 calorie; 0 g protein; 0 g carbohydrates; 0 g total fat; 0 g saturated fat; 0 g polyunsaturated fat; 0 g monounsaturated fat; 0 mg cholesterol; 0 g fiber; 4 mg sodium

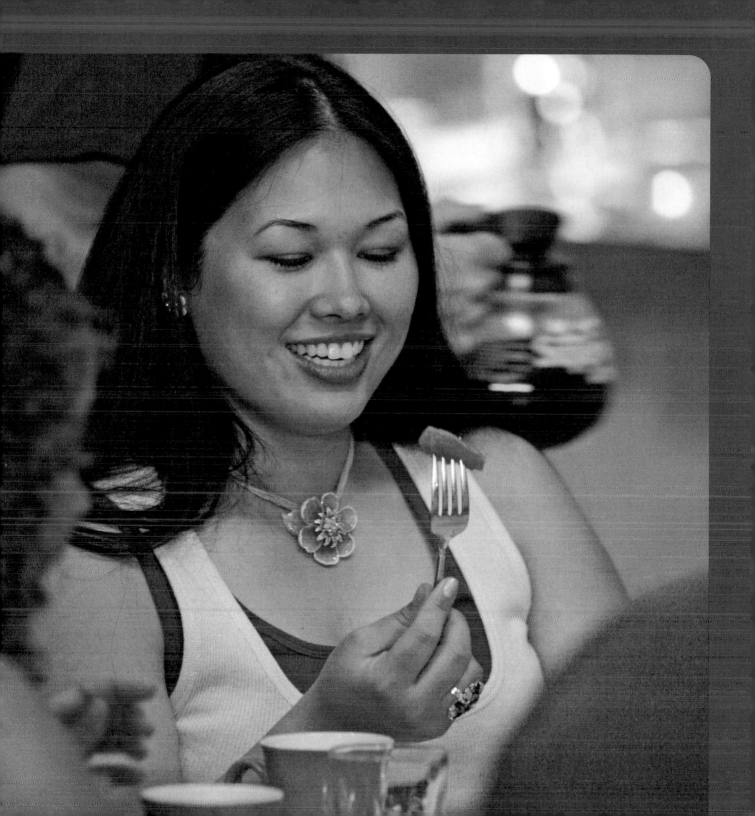

Appendix: Meal Plans

1,200-Calorie Sample Menus

day one

Breakfast

½ cup (3) egg whites scrambled with 1 teaspoon olive oil, 1 teaspoon chopped basil, 1 teaspoon grated Parmesan, and ½ cup cherry tomatoes

¾ cup fat-free milk

⅓ cup fresh blueberries

1 cup decaf iced tea with lemon

Midmorning Snack

½ cup fat-free vanilla yogurt (or frozen yogurt) sprinkled with 2 tablespoons sliced strawberries

Lunch

Southwestern bulgur salad: ½ cup cooked bulgur, 3 ounces chopped grilled chicken breast, and 1 cup diced grilled veggies (2 tablespoons onion, ¼ cup diced zucchini, ½ cup bell pepper)

1 teaspoon chopped cilantro with 1 serving (1 tablespoon) Mo Walker's Salsa Vinaigrette (page 157) and 2 teaspoons shredded low-fat Cheddar cheese

Midafternoon Snack

1 serving (2 tablespoons) Creamy Hummus (page 146) and ½ cup jicama slices

Dinner

1 serving (approximately 1 cup) Lisa Andreone's Wild Rice and Toasted Almonds (page 130)

3 ounces grilled salmon fillet

1 cup wilted baby spinach with 1 teaspoon olive oil, 1 teaspoon balsamic vinegar, and 1 teaspoon grated Parmesan cheese

½ cup diced cantaloupe

Evening Snack

1 serving (approximately ½ cup) Kathryn Murphy's Easy Raspberry Sorbet (page 155) with 1 teaspoon chopped almonds

day two

Breakfast

1 cup fresh diced melon

Oatmeal (⅓ cup dry old-fashioned oatmeal cooked with 1 tablespoon ground flax and ⅔ cup water) sprinkled with cinnamon and 2 teaspoons chopped pecans

⅓ cup fat-free vanilla yogurt

1 serving (1 cup) Mint Tea (page 158)

Midmorning Snack

1 fresh pear sliced and topped with ⅓ cup fat-free ricotta and drizzled with 1 teaspoon honey

Lunch

Mediterranean turkey pita sandwich: 1 4-inch whole wheat pita bread, 4 ounces thinly sliced lean turkey breast, ½ roasted red bell pepper, 2 pieces romaine lettuce, and 1 serving (1 tablespoon) Tangy Tahini Mustard Sauce (page 156)

Midafternoon Snack

1 fat-free mozzarella string cheese stick

1 medium tangerine

Dinner

1 serving Mark Yesitis's Grilled Italian Flank Steak with Roma Tomatoes (page 140)

Large tossed salad (2 cups mixed salad greens, ¼ cup sliced cucumbers, ¼ cup sliced mushrooms) and 1 tablespoon light Caesar dressing

Evening Snack

1 serving the Kelly Mac Snack (page 148)

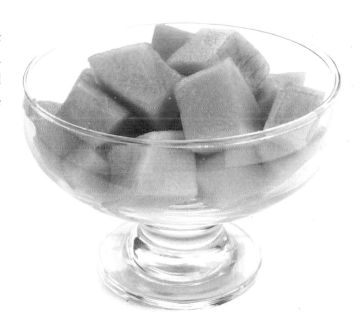

day three

Breakfast

1 cup low-sodium tomato vegetable juice

$\frac{1}{3}$ cup (2) egg whites scrambled with 1 teaspoon fresh herbs, $\frac{1}{4}$ cup chopped red onion, and $\frac{1}{4}$ cup sliced mushrooms

1 serving (2 links) Country-Style Turkey Links (page 124)

$\frac{1}{2}$ cup fresh blueberries

1 cup green tea

Midmorning Snack

1 serving (8 triangles) Ryan Kelly's Pita Triangles (page 152) and 1 serving (2 tablespoons) Creamy Hummus (page 146)

Lunch

Chicken Caesar salad: 3 ounces boneless, skinless roasted chicken, 1 cup chopped romaine lettuce, $\frac{1}{4}$ cup sliced bell pepper, $\frac{1}{4}$ cup chopped green onions, and 2 tablespoons light Caesar dressing

Midafternoon Snack

$\frac{1}{4}$ cup fat-free cottage cheese with $\frac{1}{2}$ cup tomato salsa

Dinner

1 serving Suzanne Mendonca's Grilled Salmon Burgers (page 143)

1 cup oven-roasted cauliflower and broccoli florets

$\frac{1}{2}$ cup brown rice, cooked

1 cup watercress salad with 1 tablespoon light balsamic vinaigrette

Evening Snack

$\frac{1}{4}$ cup fat-free ricotta with $\frac{1}{2}$ cup raspberries and 2 teaspoons chopped almonds

day four

Breakfast

$\frac{1}{2}$ cup diced watermelon

1 serving Aaron Semmel's Omelette of Champions (page 127)

Small quesadilla: $\frac{1}{2}$ of one small corn tortilla and 1 table-spoon low-fat Jack cheese

Iced tea with fresh lemon

Midmorning Snack

$\frac{1}{4}$ cup fat-free vanilla yogurt with $\frac{1}{2}$ sliced apple and 1 tea-spoon chopped walnuts

Lunch

1 serving Dave Fioravanti's Grilled Chicken Salad (page 131)

1 whole grain Wasa cracker

1 medium nectarine

Midafternoon Snack

$\frac{1}{2}$ serving (2 spears) Matt Kamont's Roast Asparagus with Smoked Salmon (page 149)

Dinner

3 ounces shrimp, grilled or sautéed with 1 teaspoon olive oil and 1 teaspoon chopped garlic

1 medium artichoke, steamed

$\frac{1}{2}$ cup cooked whole wheat couscous with 2 tablespoons diced bell pepper, 2 tablespoons chickpeas, 1 teaspoon chopped fresh cilantro, and 1 tablespoon fat-free honey mustard vinaigrette

Evening Snack

$\frac{1}{4}$ cup sliced strawberries with $\frac{1}{4}$ cup fat free frozen vanilla yogurt

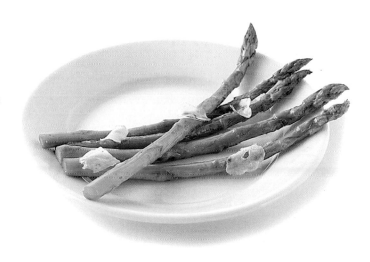

day five

Breakfast

1 serving Shannon Mullen's Egg Foo Yung (page 126)

1 wedge honeydew melon

½ slice Ezekiel bread

1 cup fat-free milk

Coffee

Midmorning Snack

Dana DeSilvio's Yogurt Parfait (page 128)

Lunch

Roast-beef wrap: 3 ounces thinly sliced lean roast beef (or chicken or turkey or pork), 1 6-inch whole wheat tortilla, ¼ cup shredded lettuce, 1 medium tomato slice, 1 teaspoon horseradish, and 1 teaspoon Dijon mustard

⅓ cup cooked pinto beans or lentils with 1 teaspoon chopped basil and 1 tablespoon light Caesar vinaigrette

Midafternoon Snack

1 serving (8 chips) Andrea Baptiste's Baked Corn Chips (page 144) with 1 serving (2 tablespoons) Edamame Guacamole (page 145)

Dinner

3 ounces grilled salmon or halibut fillet

½ cup sliced mushrooms sautéed with 1 teaspoon olive oil, ¼ cup chopped yellow onion, and ¼ cup sliced bell pepper

1 cup arugula salad with ¼ cup halved cherry tomatoes and 1 tablespoon miso dressing

Evening Snack

⅓ cup warm unsweetened applesauce with 1 tablespoon fat-free vanilla yogurt and a dash of ground cinnamon

1 serving (1 cup) Mint Tea (page 158)

day six

Breakfast

Breakfast burrito: 1 medium whole wheat tortilla, 3 scrambled egg whites, 2 tablespoons fat-free refried black beans, 2 tablespoons salsa, 1 tablespoon grated low-fat Cheddar cheese, and 1 teaspoon fresh cilantro

$\frac{1}{2}$ cup mixed melon

Iced tea

Midmorning Snack

1 serving (2 tablespoons) Jen Kersey's Peanutty Spread (page 154) and 1 medium celery stalk, cut into sticks

Lunch

1 serving Matt Hoover's Chipotle Chicken (page 151) (made with a 3-ounce chicken breast)

1 serving ($\frac{1}{2}$ cup) Barbecue Lentils (page 129)

Spinach salad: 1 cup baby spinach leaves, $\frac{1}{4}$ cup halved cherry tomatoes, 1 tablespoon light Russian vinaigrette, and 1 teaspoon grated Parmesan cheese

$\frac{3}{4}$ cup fat-free milk

Midafternoon Snack

1 fat-free mozzarella string cheese stick

$\frac{1}{4}$ cup red grapes

Dinner

1 serving Pete Thomas's Slivered Pork Stir-Fry with Garlic, Broccoli, and Sesame (page 141)

$\frac{1}{3}$ cup brown rice or bulgur wheat, cooked

3 medium tomato slices with 1 teaspoon balsamic vinegar and 1 teaspoon chopped fresh basil

Evening Snack

1 serving ($\frac{3}{4}$ cup) Banana Fudge Smoothie (page 123)

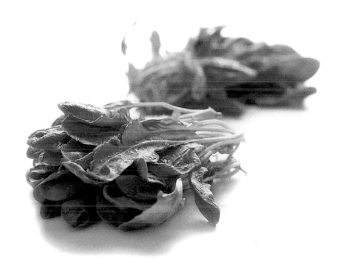

day seven

Breakfast

Breakfast frittata: $\frac{1}{2}$ cup (3 egg whites, large), 2 tablespoons diced bell peppers, 2 tablespoons chopped spinach, 1 tablespoon shredded low-fat mozzarella, and 1 teaspoon pesto

$\frac{1}{2}$ cup fat-free milk

$\frac{1}{3}$ cup fresh raspberries

1 serving (1 muffin) Blueberry Bran Mini Muffins (page 125)

Midmorning Snack

$\frac{1}{2}$ cup low-fat vanilla yogurt with 1 tablespoon ground flax and $\frac{1}{4}$ cup diced peach or pear

Lunch

2 servings Ryan Benson's Portobello "Pizzas" (page 136)

Tomato cucumber salad: 3 slices fresh tomato, $\frac{1}{4}$ cup sliced cucumber, 1 teaspoon fresh chopped thyme, and 1 tablespoon fat-free Italian dressing

1 medium orange

Midafternoon Snack

Smoothie: $\frac{1}{2}$ cup fat-free milk, $\frac{1}{2}$ banana, 3 tablespoons low-fat yogurt, and 2 tablespoons sliced strawberries

Dinner

4 ounces red snapper baked with 1 teaspoon olive oil, 1 teaspoon lemon juice, and $\frac{1}{2}$ teaspoon nonsodium seasoning

$\frac{1}{2}$ cup spaghetti squash with 1 teaspoon olive oil and 1 teaspoon grated Parmesan cheese

1 cup steamed green beans sprinkled with 2 teaspoons slivered almonds

Evening Snack

1 serving Kelly Minner's Cream Cheese Roll-Ups (page 153)

day one

Breakfast

½ cup (3) egg whites scrambled with 1 teaspoon olive oil, 1 teaspoon chopped basil, 1 teaspoon grated Parmesan cheese, and ½ cup cherry tomatoes

1 slice Ezekiel toast

1 cup fat free milk

½ cup fresh blueberries

1 cup decaf iced tea with lemon

Midmorning Snack

½ cup fat-free vanilla yogurt (or frozen yogurt) sprinkled with 2 tablespoons sliced strawberries

Lunch

Southwestern bulgur salad: ¾ cup cooked bulgur, 4 ounces chopped grilled chicken breast, and 1 cup diced grilled veggies (2 tablespoons onion, ¼ cup diced zucchini, ½ cup bell pepper)

1 teaspoon chopped cilantro with 1 serving (1 tablespoon) Mo Walker's Salsa Vinaigrette (page 157) and 1 tablespoon shredded low-fat Cheddar cheese

Midafternoon Snack

1 serving (2 tablespoons) Creamy Hummus (page 146) and ½ cup jicama slices

Dinner

1 serving (approximately 1 cup) Lisa Andreone's Wild Rice and Toasted Almonds (page 130)

4 ounces grilled salmon fillet

1 cup wilted baby spinach with 1 teaspoon olive oil, 1 teaspoon balsamic vinegar, and 1 teaspoon grated Parmesan cheese

½ cup diced cantaloupe

Evening Snack

1 serving (approximately ½ cup) Kathryn Murphy's Easy Raspberry Sorbet (page 155) with 1 teaspoon chopped almonds

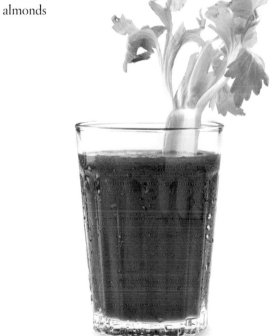

day two

Breakfast

$\frac{1}{2}$ cup fresh diced melon

Oatmeal ($\frac{1}{2}$ cup dry old-fashioned oatmeal cooked with 1 tablespoon ground flax and 1 cup water) sprinkled with cinnamon and 1 tablespoon chopped pecans

$\frac{1}{2}$ cup fat-free vanilla yogurt

1 serving (1 cup) Mint Tea (page 158)

Midmorning Snack

1 fresh pear sliced and topped with $\frac{1}{2}$ cup fat-free ricotta and drizzled with 1 teaspoon honey

Lunch

Mediterranean turkey pita sandwich: 4-inch whole wheat pita bread, 4 $\frac{1}{2}$ ounces thinly sliced lean turkey breast, $\frac{1}{2}$ roasted red bell pepper, 2 pieces romaine lettuce, and 1 serving (1 tablespoon) Tangy Tahini Mustard Sauce (page 156)

Midafternoon Snack

1 fat-free mozzarella string cheese stick

1 medium orange

Dinner

1 serving Mark Yesitis's Grilled Italian Flank Steak with Roma Tomatoes (page 140)

Large tossed salad (2 cups mixed salad greens, $\frac{1}{4}$ cup sliced cucumbers, $\frac{1}{4}$ cup sliced mushrooms) and 2 tablespoons light Caesar dressing

$\frac{3}{4}$ cup whole wheat couscous

1 cup fat-free milk

Herbal tea

Evening Snack

1 serving the Kelly Mac Snack (page 148)

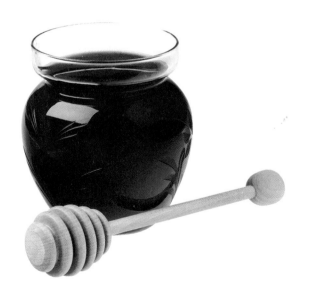

day three

Breakfast

1 cup low-sodium tomato vegetable juice

½ cup (3) egg whites scrambled with 1 teaspoon fresh herbs, ¼ cup chopped red onion, ¼ cup sliced mushrooms, and 1 tablespoon shredded low-fat Cheddar cheese

1 serving (2 links) Country-Style Turkey Links (page 124)

1 cup fresh blueberries

1 cup green tea

Midmorning Snack

1 serving (8 triangles) Ryan Kelly's Pita Triangles (page 152) and 1 serving (2 tablespoons) Creamy Hummus (page 146)

Lunch

Chicken Caesar salad: 4 ounces boneless, skinless roasted chicken, 1 cup chopped romaine lettuce, ½ cup sliced bell pepper, ¼ cup chopped green onions, and 2 tablespoons low-fat Caesar dressing

Midafternoon Snack

½ cup fat-free cottage cheese with ½ cup tomato salsa

Dinner

1 serving Suzanne Mendonca's Grilled Salmon Burgers (page 143)

1 cup oven-roasted cauliflower and broccoli florets

¾ cup brown rice, cooked

1 cup watercress salad with 1 tablespoon light balsamic vinaigrette

Evening Snack

½ cup fat-free ricotta with ½ cup raspberries and 1 tablespoon chopped almonds

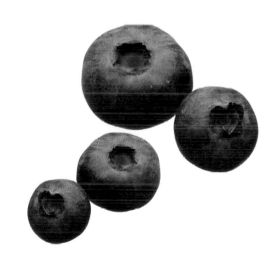

day four

Breakfast

$\frac{1}{2}$ cup diced watermelon

1 serving Aaron Semmel's Omelette of Champions (page 127)

Small quesadilla: $\frac{1}{2}$ of one small corn tortilla and 1 tablespoon low-fat Jack cheese

Iced tea with fresh lemon

Midmorning Snack

$\frac{1}{2}$ cup fat-free vanilla yogurt with 1 sliced apple and 1 tablespoon chopped walnuts

Lunch

1 serving Dave Fioravanti's Grilled Chicken Salad (page 131)

2 whole grain Wasa crackers

1 medium nectarine

Midafternoon Snack

$\frac{1}{2}$ serving (2 spears) Matt Kamont's Roast Asparagus with Smoked Salmon (page 149)

Dinner

4 ounces shrimp, grilled or sautéed with 1 teaspoon olive oil and 1 teaspoon chopped garlic

1 medium artichoke, steamed

$\frac{1}{2}$ cup cooked whole wheat couscous with 2 tablespoons diced bell pepper, $\frac{1}{4}$ cup chickpeas, 1 teaspoon chopped fresh cilantro, and 1 tablespoon fat-free honey mustard vinaigrette

Evening Snack

$\frac{1}{2}$ cup sliced strawberries with $\frac{1}{2}$ cup fat-free frozen vanilla yogurt

day five

Breakfast

1 serving Shannon Mullen's Egg Foo Yung (page 126)

1 wedge honeydew melon

1 slice Ezekiel bread, toasted

1 cup fat-free milk

Coffee

Midmorning Snack

Dana DeSilvio's Yogurt Parfait (page 128)

Lunch

Roast-beef wrap: 1 6-inch whole wheat tortilla, 4 ounces thinly sliced lean roast beef (or chicken or turkey or pork), ¼ cup shredded lettuce, 3 medium tomato slices, 1 teaspoon horseradish, 1 teaspoon Dijon mustard, and ½ cup jicama sticks

½ cup cooked pinto beans or lentils with 1 teaspoon chopped basil and 1 tablespoon light Caesar vinaigrette

Midafternoon Snack

1 serving (8 chips) Andrea Baptiste's Baked Corn Chips (page 144) with 1 serving (2 tablespoons) Edamame Guacamole (page 145)

Dinner

4 ounces grilled salmon or halibut fillet

½ cup sliced mushrooms sautéed with 1 teaspoon olive oil, ¼ cup chopped yellow onion, and ¼ cup sliced bell pepper

1 cup arugula salad with ½ cup halved cherry tomatoes and 1 tablespoon miso dressing

Evening Snack

½ cup warm unsweetened applesauce with ¼ cup fat-free vanilla yogurt, dash cinnamon, and 1 tablespoon chopped pecans

1 serving (1 cup) Mint Tea (page 158)

day six

Breakfast

Breakfast burrito: 1 medium whole wheat tortilla, ⅓ cup (4) scrambled egg whites, 1 teaspoon olive oil, ¼ cup fat-free refried black beans, 2 tablespoons salsa, 2 tablespoons grated low-fat Cheddar cheese, and 1 teaspoon fresh cilantro

1 cup mixed melon

Iced tea

Midmorning Snack

1 serving (2 tablespoons) Jen Kersey's Peanutty Spread (page 154) and 1 medium celery stalk, cut into sticks

Lunch

1 serving Matt Hoover's Chipotle Chicken (page 151) (made with a 4-ounce chicken breast)

1 serving (½ cup) Barbecue Lentils (page 129)

Spinach salad: 1 cup baby spinach leaves, ¼ cup halved cherry tomatoes, 1 tablespoon light Russian vinaigrette, and 2 teaspoons grated Parmesan cheese

1 cup fat-free milk

Midafternoon Snack

1 fat-free mozzarella string cheese stick

1 cup red grapes

Dinner

1 serving Pete Thomas's Slivered Pork Stir-Fry with Garlic, Broccoli, and Sesame (page 141)

½ cup brown rice or bulgur wheat, cooked

5 medium tomato slices with 1 teaspoon balsamic vinegar and 1 teaspoon chopped fresh basil

Evening Snack

1 serving (¾ cup) Banana Fudge Smoothie (page 123)

day seven

Breakfast

Breakfast frittata: ½ cup (3 large) egg whites, 2 tablespoons diced bell peppers, 2 tablespoons chopped spinach, 2 tablespoons low-fat shredded mozzarella, and 2 teaspoons pesto

1 cup fat-free milk

½ cup fresh raspberries

2 servings (2 muffins) Blueberry Bran Mini Muffins (page 125)

Midmorning Snack

½ cup low-fat vanilla yogurt with 1 tablespoon ground flax and ½ cup diced peach or pear

Lunch

2 servings Ryan Benson's Portobello "Pizzas" (page 136)

Tomato cucumber salad: 5 slices fresh tomato, ¼ cup sliced cucumber, 1 teaspoon fresh chopped thyme, and 1 tablespoon fat-free Italian dressing

1 medium orange

Midafternoon Snack

Smoothie made with ¾ cup fat-free milk, ½ banana, ½ cup low-fat yogurt, and ¼ cup sliced strawberries

Dinner

4 ounces red snapper baked with 1 teaspoon olive oil, 1 teaspoon lemon juice, and ½ teaspoon nonsodium seasoning

1 cup spaghetti squash with 1 teaspoon olive oil and 2 teaspoons grated Parmesan cheese

1 cup steamed green beans sprinkled with 1 tablespoon slivered almonds

Evening Snack

1 serving Kelly Minner's Cream Cheese Roll-Ups (page 153)

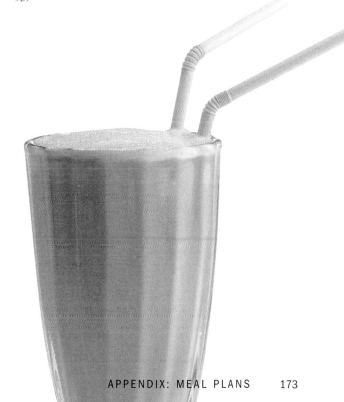

day one

Breakfast

4 large egg whites scrambled with 1 teaspoon olive oil, 1 teaspoon chopped basil, 1 teaspoon grated Parmesan cheese, and ½ cup cherry tomatoes

1 slice Ezekiel toast

1 cup fat-free milk

½ cup fresh blueberries

1 cup decaf iced tea with lemon

Midmorning Snack

¾ cup fat-free vanilla yogurt (or frozen yogurt) sprinkled with ¼ cup sliced strawberries

Lunch

Southwestern bulgur salad: 1 cup cooked bulgur, 5 ounces chopped grilled chicken breast, and 1½ cups diced grilled veggies (¼ cup chopped onion, ¾ cup diced zucchini, ½ cup bell pepper)

1 teaspoon chopped cilantro with 2 servings (2 tablespoons) Mo Walker's Salsa Vinaigrette (page 157) and 2 tablespoons shredded low-fat Cheddar cheese

Midafternoon Snack

1 serving (2 tablespoons) Creamy Hummus (page 146) and ½ cup jicama slices

Dinner

1 serving (approximately 1 cup) Lisa Andreone's Wild Rice and Toasted Almonds (page 130)

5 ounces grilled salmon fillet

1½ cups wilted baby spinach with 1 teaspoon olive oil, 1 teaspoon balsamic vinegar, and 1 tablespoon grated Parmesan cheese

1 cup diced cantaloupe

Evening Snack

1 serving (approximately ½ cup) Kathryn Murphy's Easy Raspberry Sorbet (page 155) with 1 tablespoon chopped almonds

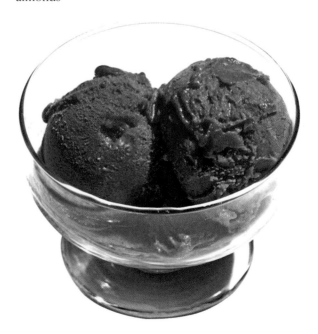

day two

Breakfast

1 cup fresh diced melon

Oatmeal ($\frac{1}{2}$ cup dry old-fashioned oatmeal cooked with 1 tablespoon ground flax and 1 cup water) sprinkled with cinnamon and 1 tablespoon chopped pecans

$\frac{1}{2}$ cup fat-free vanilla yogurt

1 serving (1 cup) Mint Tea (page 158)

Midmorning Snack

$\frac{1}{2}$ fresh pear sliced and topped with $\frac{1}{2}$ cup fat-free ricotta and drizzled with 1 teaspoon honey

Lunch

Mediterranean turkey pita sandwich: 1 4-inch whole wheat pita bread, $4\frac{1}{2}$ ounces thinly sliced lean turkey breast, $\frac{1}{2}$ roasted red bell pepper, 2 pieces romaine lettuce, 1 serving (1 tablespoon) Tangy Tahini Mustard Sauce (page 156)

Midafternoon Snack

1 fat-free mozzarella string cheese stick

1 medium orange

Dinner

1 serving Mark Yesitis's Grilled Italian Flank Steak with Roma Tomatoes (page 140)

Large tossed salad (2 cups mixed salad greens, $\frac{1}{4}$ cup sliced cucumbers, $\frac{1}{4}$ cup sliced mushrooms) and 2 tablespoons light Caesar dressing

$\frac{3}{4}$ cup whole wheat couscous

$\frac{3}{4}$ cup fat-free milk

Herbal tea

Evening Snack

1 serving the Kelly Mac Snack (page 148)

day three

Breakfast

1 cup low-sodium tomato vegetable juice

½ cup (3) egg whites scrambled with 1 teaspoon olive oil, 1 teaspoon fresh herbs, ¼ cup chopped red onion, ¼ cup sliced mushrooms, and 1 tablespoon shredded low-fat Cheddar cheese

1½ servings (3 links) Country-Style Turkey Links (page 124)

1 cup fresh blueberries

1 cup green tea

Midmorning Snack

1 serving (8 triangles) Ryan Kelly's Pita Triangles (page 152) and 1 serving (2 tablespoons) Creamy Hummus (page 146)

Lunch

Chicken Caesar salad: 5 ounces boneless, skinless roasted chicken, 1 cup chopped romaine lettuce, ½ cup sliced bell pepper, ¼ cup chopped green onions, and 2 tablespoons low-fat Caesar dressing

Midafternoon Snack

½ cup fat-free cottage cheese with ½ cup tomato salsa

Dinner

1 serving Suzanne Mendonca's Grilled Salmon Burgers (page 143)

1 cup oven-roasted cauliflower and broccoli florets

1 cup brown rice, cooked

1 cup watercress salad with 1 tablespoon light balsamic vinaigrette

1 cup fat-free milk

Evening Snack

½ cup fat-free ricotta with ¾ cup raspberries and 1 tablespoon chopped almonds

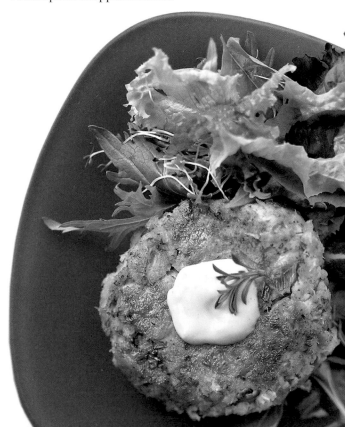

day four

Breakfast

$1/2$ cup diced watermelon

1 serving Aaron Semmel's Omelette of Champions (page 127)

Small quesadilla: 1 small corn tortilla and 2 tablespoons low-fat Jack cheese

Iced tea with fresh lemon

Midmorning Snack

$3/4$ cup fat-free vanilla yogurt with 1 sliced apple and 1 tablespoon chopped walnuts

Lunch

1 serving Dave Fioravanti's Grilled Chicken Salad (page 131)

2 whole grain Wasa crackers

1 medium nectarine

Midafternoon Snack

1 serving (4 spears) Matt Kamont's Roast Asparagus with Smoked Salmon (page 149)

Dinner

5 ounces shrimp, grilled or sautéed with 1 teaspoon olive oil and 1 teaspoon chopped garlic

1 medium artichoke, steamed

$1/2$ cup cooked whole wheat couscous with 2 tablespoons diced bell pepper, 3 tablespoons chickpeas, 1 teaspoon chopped fresh cilantro, and 1 tablespoon fat-free honey mustard vinaigrette

Evening Snack

$1/2$ cup sliced strawberries with $3/4$ cup fat-free frozen vanilla yogurt

day five

Breakfast

1 serving Shannon Mullen's Egg Foo Yung (page 126)

1 cup diced melon and ¼ cup blueberries with 1 teaspoon fresh mint

1 slice Ezekiel bread, toasted

1 cup fat-free milk

Coffee

Midmorning Snack

Dana DeSilvio's Yogurt Parfait (page 128)

Lunch

Roast-beef wrap: 1 6-inch whole wheat tortilla, 5 ounces thinly sliced lean roast beef (or chicken or turkey or pork), ¼ cup shredded lettuce, 3 medium tomato slices, 1 teaspoon horseradish, 1 teaspoon Dijon mustard, and ¾ cup jicama sticks

¾ cup cooked pinto beans or lentils with 1 teaspoon chopped basil and 1 tablespoon light Caesar vinaigrette

Midafternoon Snack

1½ servings (12 chips) Andrea Baptiste's Baked Corn Chips (page 144) with 1½ servings (3 tablespoons) Edamame Guacamole (page 145)

Dinner

5½ ounces grilled salmon or halibut fillet

½ cup sliced mushrooms sautéed with 1 teaspoon olive oil, ¼ cup chopped yellow onion, and ½ cup sliced bell pepper

1½ cups arugula salad with ½ cup halved cherry tomatoes and 2 tablespoons miso dressing

Evening Snack

¾ cup warm unsweetened applesauce with ½ cup fat-free vanilla yogurt, dash cinnamon, and 1 tablespoon chopped pecans

1 serving (1 cup) Mint Tea (page 158)

day six

Breakfast

Breakfast burrito: 1 medium whole wheat tortilla, ½ cup (3) scrambled egg whites , 1 teaspoon olive oil, ¼ cup fat-free refried black beans, 2 tablespoons salsa, 1 tablespoon grated low-fat Cheddar cheese, and 1 teaspoon fresh cilantro

1 cup mixed melon

⅓ cup fat-free vanilla yogurt

Iced tea

Midmorning Snack

1 serving (2 tablespoons) Jen Kersey's Peanutty Spread (page 154) and 1 medium celery stalk, cut into sticks

Lunch

1serving Matt Hoover's Chipotle Chicken (page 151) (made with a 6-ounce chicken breast)

1 serving (½ cup) Barbecue Lentils (page 129)

Spinach salad: 1½ cups baby spinach leaves, ¼ cup halved cherry tomatoes, 2 tablespoons light Russian vinaigrette, and 2 teaspoons grated Parmesan cheese

1 cup fat-free milk

Midafternoon Snack

1 fat-free mozzarella string cheese stick

¾ cup red grapes

Dinner

1 serving Pete Thomas's Slivered Pork Stir-Fry with Garlic, Broccoli, and Sesame (page 141)

½ cup brown rice or bulgur wheat, cooked

3 medium tomato slices with 1 teaspoon balsamic vinegar and 1 teaspoon chopped fresh basil

1 medium pear

Green tea

Evening Snack

1 serving (¾ cup) Banana Fudge Smoothie (page 123)

11 almonds

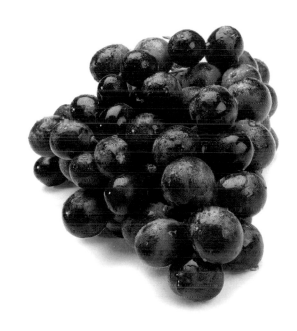

day seven

Breakfast

Breakfast frittata: $\frac{1}{2}$ cup (3 large) egg whites, 2 tablespoons diced bell peppers, 2 tablespoons chopped spinach, 2 tablespoons shredded low-fat mozzarella, and 2 teaspoons pesto

2 soy sausage patties

1 cup fat-free milk

$\frac{1}{2}$ cup fresh raspberries

2 servings (2 muffins) Blueberry Bran Mini Muffins (page 125)

Midmorning Snack

$\frac{1}{2}$ cup fat-free vanilla yogurt with 1 tablespoon ground flax and $\frac{1}{2}$ cup diced peach or pear

Lunch

2 servings Ryan Benson's Portobello "Pizzas" (page 136)

Tomato cucumber salad: 4 slices fresh tomato, $\frac{1}{4}$ cup sliced cucumber, 1 teaspoon fresh chopped thyme, and 1 tablespoon fat-free Italian dressing

1 medium orange

Midafternoon Snack

Smoothie: $\frac{3}{4}$ cup fat-free milk, $\frac{1}{2}$ medium banana, $\frac{1}{2}$ cup low-fat yogurt, and $\frac{1}{4}$ cup sliced strawberries

1 whole grain Wasa cracker with 2 teaspoons creamy peanut butter

Dinner

5 ounces red snapper baked with 1 teaspoon olive oil, 1 teaspoon lemon juice, and $\frac{1}{2}$ teaspoon nonsodium seasoning

$\frac{3}{4}$ cup spaghetti squash with 1 teaspoon olive oil and 2 teaspoons grated Parmesan cheese

$\frac{1}{2}$ cup steamed green beans sprinkled with 1 tablespoon slivered almonds

Evening Snack

1 serving Kelly Minner's Cream Cheese Roll-Ups (page 153)

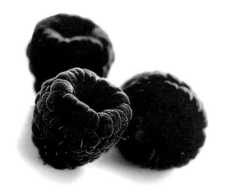

Contributors

Bob Harper, trainer on *The Biggest Loser*, is one of America's favorite trainers and counts Gwyneth Paltrow, Ben Stiller, and Ellen DeGeneres among his past and present clients. He recently worked with Sam Mendes on *Jarhead*, training the cast to get into shape to portray Marines. His favorite activities include tennis, cycling, snowboarding, kickboxing, and yoga. He is an avid runner and has completed two marathons; he also enjoys photography and reading. He lives in Los Angeles.

Jillian Michaels, trainer on *The Biggest Loser*, holds personal training certificates from the National Endurance and Strength Training Association (NESTA) and the American Fitness Association of America (AFAA). Her celebrity clientele includes entertainment mogul David Geffen, Amanda Peet, Vanessa Marcil, Amber Tamblyn, Jeremy Rener, and Sarah Paulson. She lives in Los Angeles.

Michael Dansinger, MD, is the director of the Tufts Popular Diet Trial, a widely publicized study comparing the effects of the Atkins, Zone, Weight Watchers, and Ornish diets for weight loss and heart disease prevention. A leading authority on popular diets and weight loss, he lectures to medical and nonmedical audiences throughout the United States. He directs a weight-loss practice and research program in Boston.

Cheryl Forberg, RD, consulting dietitian to *The Biggest Loser*, earned her degree in nutrition and clinical dietetics from the University of California at Berkeley. Cheryl is a food and nutrition journalist, a James Beard award-winning recipe developer, and author of *Stop the Clock! Cooking: Defy Aging—Eat the Foods You Love* (Avery-Penguin Group).

Maggie Greenwood-Robinson, PhD, is a leading health and medical writer in the United States. She has authored or coauthored more than 30 books on nutrition, exercise, weight loss, brain fitness, and health issues such as cancer. Among her most recent books are *Good Carbs versus Bad Carbs* and *The Bikini Diet*. She has a doctorate in nutritional counseling.

The Biggest Loser Cast: Season One

Lisa Andreone

Andrea Baptiste

Ryan Benson

Lizzeth Davalos

Gary Deckman

Dana DeSilvio

David Fioravanti

Matt Kamont

Kelly MacFarland

Kelly Minner

Aaron Semmel

Maurice Walker

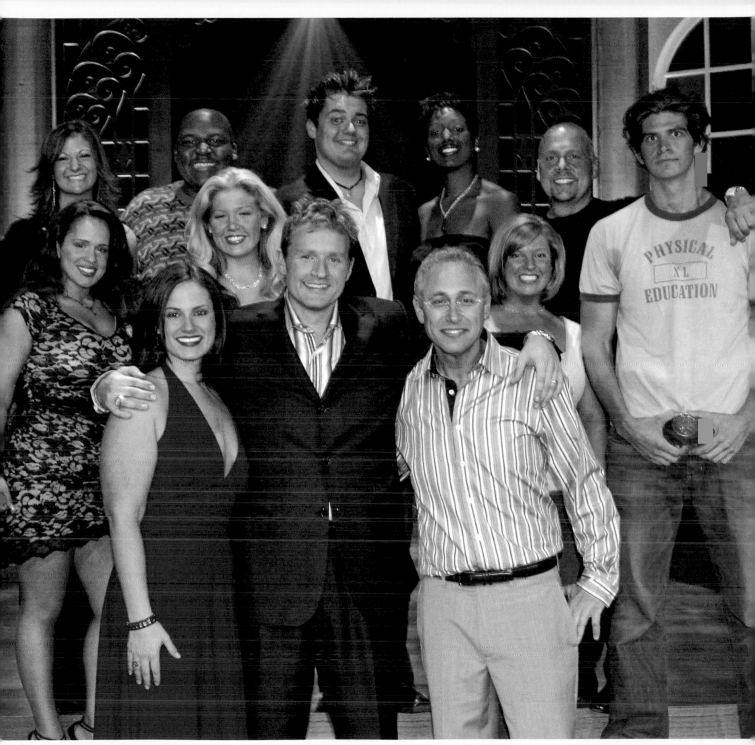

Season one cast at the end

The Biggest Loser Cast: Season Two

Nick Gaza

Ruben Hernandez

Matt Hoover

Ryan Kelly

Jen Kersey

Jeff Levine

Suzanne Mendonca

Shannon Mullen

Kathryn Murphy

Andrea Overstreet

Suzy Preston

Pete Thomas

Seth Word

Mark Yesitis

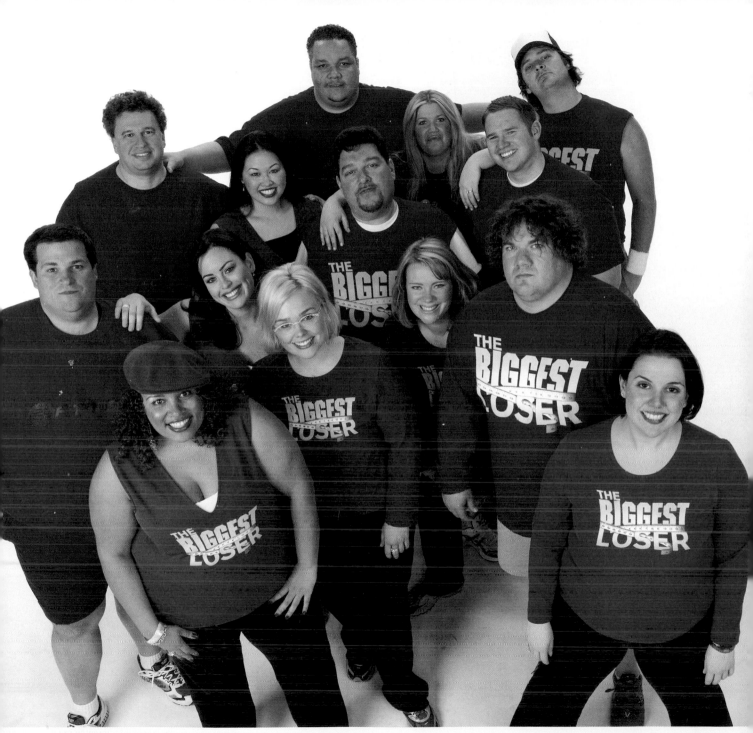

Season two cast at the beginning

Index

Boldface page references indicate photographs and illustrations. <u>Underscored</u> references indicate boxed text.

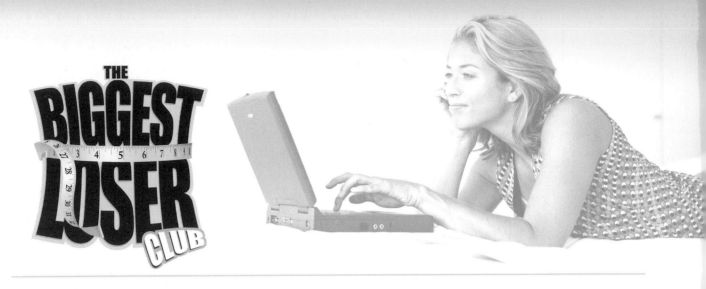

Make your goals even easier to reach...
become part of The Biggest Loser Club!

If you're serious about making a real change in your life, you won't want to miss your chance to explore The Biggest Loser Club risk-free. This revolutionary site allows you to design and implement the perfect program to reach your health goals, whether you're looking to lose 10 pounds or 100 pounds. Join other people, just like you, striving to make a satisfying change in their lives, and achieve the body you've longed for once and for all!

Start by enjoying a RISK-FREE TRIAL, with access to <u>everything</u>:

- **Personalize your own Online Diet** and Fitness Program
- **Create an online journal** to track your own results
- **Find tons of delicious, healthy recipes** you won't find in the book
- **Visit the community forums** to share tips and advice and to stay motivated
- **Exclusive updates and access** to The Biggest Loser trainers and contestants
- **FREE Biggest Loser Club weekly e-newsletter** included

As seen on

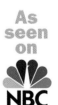

NBC

Only at www.biggestloserclub.com/book
Check it out—RISK-FREE—today!

See how easy it can be...take the **Free Tour** at the Web site above to learn more.

200565301